Practical Manual of Abdominal Organ Transplantation

Practical Manual of Abdominal Organ Transplantation

Edited by

Cosme Manzarbeitia, M.D.
Albert Einstein Medical Center
Philadelphia, Pennsylvania

Kluwer Academic / Plenum Publishers
New York   Boston   London   Dordrecht   Moscow

Library of Congress Cataloging-in-Publication Data

Practical manual of abdominal organ transplantation/edited by
Cosme Manzarbeitia
   p.   ; cm.
Includes bibliographical references and index.
ISBN 0-306-46639-2
   1. Transplantation of organs, tissues, etc.—Handbooks,
manuals, etc.   2. Abdomen—Surgery—Handbooks, manuals, etc.   3.
Liver—Transplantation—Handbooks, manuals, etc.
   [DNLM: 1. Liver Transplantation—Handbooks.   2. Kidney
Transplantation—Handbooks.   3. Pancreas
Transplantation—Handbooks.   WI 39 P895 2002]   I. Manzarbeitia,
Cosme, 1959–
   RD540 .P837 2002
   617.5'50592—dc21

2001053921

ISBN: 0-306-46639-2

© 2002 Kluwer Academic / Plenum Publishers, New York
233 Spring Street, New York, New York 10013

http://www.wkap.nl

10   9 8 7 6 5 4 3 2 1

Printed in the United States of America

Contributors

Sergio Alvarez, Albert Einstein Medical Center, Philadelphia, Pennsylvania 19141

Victor Araya, Albert Einstein Medical Center, Philadelphia, Pennsylvania 19141

Ierachmiel Daskal, Albert Einstein Medical Center, Philadelphia, Pennsylvania 19141

Sukru Emre, Mount Sinai Medical Center, New York, New York 10029

Javid Fazili, Albert Einstein Medical Center, Philadelphia, Pennsylvania 19141

Arthur J. Geller, Freehold, New Jersey 07728

Kevin Hails, Albert Einstein Medical Center, Philadelphia, Pennsylvania 19141

Steven-Huy Han, UCLA School of Medicine, Los Angeles, California 90095

Vivek Kaul, Albert Einstein Medical Center, Philadelphia, Pennsylvania 19141

Jan Kramer, Albert Einstein Medical Center, Philadelphia, Pennsylvania 19141

Laurel Lerner, Albert Einstein Medical Center, Philadelphia, Pennsylvania 19141

Michael K. McGuire, Albert Einstein Medical Center, Philadelphia, Pennsylvania 19141

Cosme Manzarbeitia, Albert Einstein Medical Center, Philadelphia, Pennsylvania 19141

Paul Martin, UCLA School of Medicine, Los Angeles, California 90095

Rohit Moghe, Albert Einstein Medical Center, Philadelphia, Pennsylvania 19141

M. Catherine Morrison, Albert Einstein Medical Center, Philadelphia, Pennsylvania 19141

Santiago J. Munoz, Albert Einstein Medical Center, Philadelphia, Pennsylvania 19141

Juan Oleaga, Albert Einstein Medical Center, Philadelphia, Pennsylvania 19141

Jorge A. Ortiz, Albert Einstein Medical Center, Philadelphia, Pennsylvania 19141

Lloyd E. Ratner, Johns Hopkins University School of Medicine, Baltimore, Maryland 21287

David J. Reich, Albert Einstein Medical Center, Philadelphia, Pennsylvania 19141

Jonathan V. Roth, Albert Einstein Medical Center, Philadelphia, Pennsylvania 19141

Kenneth D. Rothstein, Albert Einstein Medical Center, Philadelphia, Pennsylvania 19141

Sammy Saab, UCLA School of Medicine, Los Angeles, California 90095

Henkie P. Tan, Johns Hopkins University School of Medicine, Baltimore, Maryland 21287

Shuin-Lin Yang, Albert Einstein Medical Center, Philadelphia, Pennsylvania 19141

Nayere Zaeri, Albert Einstein Medical Center, Philadelphia, Pennsylvania 19141

Radi Zaki, Albert Einstein Medical Center, Philadelphia, Pennsylvania 19141

Preface

Replacement of diseased tissue with new, healthy tissue is not a new dream. Mankind entertained this idea since even before written history, the concept of repair and replacement of body portions being quite prevalent in the lore of primitive people. Legend speaks of the saints, Cosmas and Damian, transplanting a gangrenous leg from one human to another. In medieval times, belief in magical powers began to decline as resurgence in the investigative spirit took precedence. In the nineteenth century, John Hunter performed ample experiments in autografting solid organ fragments. At the same time, a renewed interest in plastic surgical procedures led to several key discoveries, such as the temperature and neo-vascularization dependence of grafts.

The development of vascular surgery in the early 1990s paved the way for successful organ revascularization. Jaboulay and Unger were the first to attempt vascularized xenografts in humans. Alexis Carrel further developed modern vascular techniques and established the need for core cooling of grafts. Simultaneously, work had begun earlier in the field of immunology on the theories of histocompatibility. Rejection mechanisms were more clearly understood after the classic observations of Medawar and Gibson in the 1940s, which gave way to the discovery of the cellular component of the rejection mechanism, paved the way for immunologic tolerance theories and studies, and brought the role of the lymphocyte to the forefront as an immunocompetent cell. In the 1950s, Hume in Boston, and Kuss in Paris, further developed kidney transplantation, which would see a large-scale resurgence in 1960. In 1952, Jean Dausset described the major histocompatibility complex genes in humans, and in 1954, Joseph Murray performed the first successful human kidney transplant, which later won him the Nobel Prize. However, the rate of graft loss was still very high due to rejection, which led to attempts to modify the immune response to promote graft acceptance. The discovery and use of 6-mercaptopurine (6-MP) and its derivatives by Calne and Murray gave poor results until combined later with steroids by Starzl and others. The results of kidney transplantation slowly improved and technical advances were made, along with the discovery of transplant-associated complications, such as hyperacute rejection from preformed antibodies, emergence of infections and tumors, and the long-term effects of steroids. Tissue typing also developed during the 1960s, with further clarification of the role of human leukocyte antigens (HLAs). Also in this decade, brain death criteria were established and newer preservation solutions were developed, specifically, the solution by Folkert Belzer in 1967 at the University of Wisconsin. This stimulated the first attempts at transplant of other organs, such as liver (Starzl, 1963), lung (Hardy, 1963), heart (Barnard, 1967) and pancreas (Lillehei, 1966). The 1970s brought about a flurry of curiosity and maturation in the kidney transplant arena, followed by further developments in the other organ transplant systems (heart, liver, lung, and pancreas). Though considerable ethical issues remained, work on the definition of brain death, which had started in 1968, led to practical use of guidelines in the mid-1970s. Azathioprine, a 6-MP derivative, and steroids were the unchallenged standard combination of immunosuppressive drugs used until cyclosporine emerged in 1979, making transplantation safer and more successful. The 1980s brought about an immense growth in transplantation thanks to cyclosporine, and, as experience was gained in its use, results improved. Concomitant advances in detection of rejection and infections such as cytomegalovirus (CMV) were also substantial. More recent developments that have brought us into the 21st century include newer immunosuppressive agents, such as tacrolimus, receptor-aimed monoclonal and polyclonal antibodies, mycophenolate, and sirolimus. The latest approaches being evaluated include the search for consistent tolerance induction, the Holy Grail of transplantation. In summary, within the last four decades, transplantation of solid organs has evolved from an experimental surgical *tour de force* to an accepted, scientifically sound modality of treatment for a selected group of patients with end-stage organ disease.

At a growing number of centers in the United States and worldwide, transplant procedures now achieve 1-year survival rates greater than 80% with many long-term survivors. Many patients so transplanted lead a high-quality, economically productive life in lieu of near certain death or disability. This growth has brought about the development of transplantation programs.

While cost considerations have played a role in slowing the activation of programs (costs are in the range of $60,000 to $250,000, depending on the specific organ), these figures do not accurately reflect the cost of this procedure to society. Management of end-stage organ disease is far more costly and does not yield a viable patient in the end. Optimal comparative data are not available for liver transplants. However, kidney transplantation is more cost-efficient than dialysis. The net cost of a strategy that attempts to save lives and rehabilitate patients to a level of economic viability may be only marginally greater than the current costs of terminal care, and offset by the return of the patient to society and gainful employment. The major constraint to meeting the demand for transplants is the availability of donated (cadaver) organs. Several steps have been taken, nationally and locally, to alleviate the organ shortage. National required request laws mandate that families of every medically suitable potential donor be offered the option to donate organs and tissues. In addition, laws such as Act 102, enacted in Pennsylvania, that require all deaths to be reported to organ procurement organizations (OPOs), resulting in increased organ donations, will soon be adopted nationwide. Rising public awareness about organ transplantation should continue to reduce the organ shortage. Finally, aggressive use of extended donors, reduced-size, split, and living-related liver transplantation continue to expand the organ donor pool. These efforts, however, still fail to meet the need.

In terms of procurement, allocation, and distribution, major improvements are being made nationally to optimize distribution and ensure good matches. Entry into the waiting list is being standardized by the recent development of listing criteria for all degrees of sickness. The United Network for Organ Sharing (UNOS, Richmond, Virginia) maintains a computerized registry of all patients waiting for organ transplants, and allocation is based upon degree of illness and waiting time. This organization develops and maintains the national Organ Procurement and Transplantation Network (OPTN), which in turn, is funded by the Health Resources and Services Administration (HRSA), an agency of the U.S. Department of Health and Human Services (DHHS).

As this brief historical synopsis illustrates, intra-abdominal organ transplantation has experienced vertiginous growth over the last two decades. When I first became involved in transplantation in 1989, as the first multiorgan transplant fellow of the Mount Sinai Hospital in New York City, the experience was one of the highlights of my existence. I still vividly remember my interview with my mentor, Charles Miller, a great surgeon to whom I am indebted, and my wonderful experience there. Over the years, this enthusiasm has not declined; in fact, it continues to grow strong. Perhaps motivated by this drive, I noticed that in those early times there was a need for a general, academically oriented, standardized introduction manual for those health care professionals involved with these very complex patients. This need became even more evident as I developed the multiorgan transplant program at Inova Fairfax Hospital, Virginia, from 1991 to 1995. I noticed that many physicians and nursing staff were new to intra-abdominal transplantation, and no readily available concise references existed. Though this problem had been partially overcome at the time of my move to the Albert Einstein Medical Center in Philadelphia, I resolved to develop a standard manual that could grow and develop along with the specialty, one that was large enough to be really useful and small enough to be easily portable for residents and fellows alike. Thus, this manual was born as a quick, reasonably comprehensive reference for the residents, fellows, medical students, nurses physician assistants, practicing physicians, and any other ancillary health care personnel who may interact with organ transplant recipients or simply want to enhance their knowledge of the subject.

This manual covers not only the basic concepts but also addresses other controversial and ethical topics in detailed, albeit succinct manner. Strict attention to detail and protocols, a sound clinical and surgical base, and a strong sense of teamwork will continue to make improvements in the teaching of our fellows and the success in the management of our patients. We only hope that incorporating the principles outlined herein will benefit us as well as our patients. This manual systematically goes through the same steps these patients experience, namely, workup and evaluation, management during the waiting period, the process of organ allocation, the surgical procedure, early and late complications, immunosuppression medications and side effects, and outcomes. In addition, diagnostic techniques used in the specialty are discussed. We believe that such a concise approach is beneficial in providing the reader with a practical approach to the topic, and if further in-depth analysis is required, a suggested reading section can be found at the end of this manual. Transplantation is an ever-growing, dynamic, and exciting field that offers cure possibilities to those patients suffering from end-stage organ disease. Developments continue to flourish and the only frontier at the present time seems to be the availability of transplantable cadaver organs. Once this is conquered and costs are made reasonable, the possibilities are endless.

The purpose of this manual is to familiarize the user with the most current protocols and practical issues arising in the day-to-day management of abdominal organ transplant recipients, including, but not limited to, liver, kidney, and pancreas transplantation. For an in-depth review of any given topics, the journals and textbooks listed should be consulted. Finally, practitioners should always keep in mind that no protocol is meant to be a substitute for sound clinical judgment and should exercise their own discretion for any given patient.

We are in deep gratitude to all our colleagues who have contributed to this manual, and we look forward to expanding the topics and editions as the specialty evolves in the new millennium.

ACKNOWLEDGMENTS

An old Castilian proverb translates as follows:

To be a man, one has to do three things in life:
Plant a tree, have a child, and write a book.

It is therefore only right that I thank all those responsible for who I am today.

My parents, for planting the tree of wisdom and giving me the strength and means to succeed in life.

My wife, JoAnn, for her faith, patience, and care of our children, Robert Daniel, and Aaron Joseph, who make life worth living.

My friends and colleagues, for nurturing, teaching, and helping me from my early days in Madrid to the present times.

Contents

II. ORGAN PROCUREMENT AND PRESERVATION

V. LAST POSTOPERATIVE COMPLICATIONS AND OUTCOMES

Part **I**

Pretransplant Evaluation and Management

Chapter **1**

Indications for Liver Transplantation

Victor Araya, Javid Fazili, Vivek Kaul, Kenneth D. Robinson, and Santiago J. Munoz

Selection and timing of patient referral for liver transplant (LT) evaluation is important to optimize outcomes. The worse the decompensated liver disease, the higher the perioperative mortality. Thus, patients should ideally be referred for LT evaluation before they become debilitated and develop life-threatening complications. And, by implication, it is even more important to expeditiously refer for LT, even after the patient has decompensated, because significant improvements in mortality may still be possible.

1.1. GENERAL INDICATIONS FOR LIVER TRANSPLANTATION

The indications for LT may be divided into three general categories: biochemical, clinical, and quality-of-life indications. The biochemical indications vary depending on whether liver disease is hepatocellular or cholestatic in nature. In general, referral should be considered when serum bilirubin is > 3 mg/dl, prothrombin time is prolonged > 5 seconds, or serum albumin is < 2.5 gm/dl.

Clinical criteria include progressive hepatic encephalopathy, refractory ascites, recurrent variceal bleeding, multiple episodes of spontaneous bacterial peritonitis, and intractable pruritus. Patients with refractory ascites have approximately 50% six-month and 25% one-year survival. Transjugular intrahepatic portosystemic shunt (TIPS) cn improve refractory ascites and may delay the need for LT or serve as a "bridge" to transplantation. Although a single episode of variceal bleeding is not an indication for LT, the reported 70% risk of recurrent variceal bleeding within 2 years of the index hemorrhage, with a mortality rate of 50% for each bleeding episode, suggests that LT should be seriously considered after the first variceal bleed.

Quality-of-life indications for LT include intractable pruritus, frequent episodes of bacterial cholangitis, osteoporotic fractures, and disabling fatigue. These complications, which may be present in many chronic liver diseases to some extent, can be the dominant problem in patients with cholestatic liver disease.

1.2. DISEASE-SPECIFIC INDICATIONS FOR LIVER TRANSPLANTATION

1.2.1. Acute Liver Failure

Fulminant hepatic failure (FHF) is defined as acute liver failure complicated by encephalopathy in patients with no evidence of previous liver disease. Despite maximal medical supportive therapy, mortality rates in FHF approach 75%, depending on the cause of liver injury. Artificial liver support systems are currently experimental, undergoing controlled evaluations. In patients with FHF, the results of urgent LT have been remarkable. The evaluation of a patient with FHF for urgent LT depends on careful assessment of the prognosis for survival without LT. O'Grady and colleagues at the King's College Liver Unit (*Gastroenterology* 1989;*97*:439–445) found that the most important variables predicting prognosis included patient age, disease etiology, encephalopathy grade, duration of jaundice, admission serum bilirubin level, and prothrombin time. In patients with acetaminophen-induced FHF, arterial pH on admission and serum creatinine level were closely associated with prognosis. When the King's College criteria are present, they can generally be considered indications for urgent LT. When these criteria are not met, however, the predictive value for spontaneous recovery is low. Thus, other prognostic factors are needed to improve the decision-making process for LT in patients with FHF.

1.2.2. Primary Biliary Cirrhosis (PBC)

PBC has a relatively predictable natural history and accurate prognostic models. The most important variable, common to all prognostic models, is the serum total bilirubin level. Shapiro et al. (*Gut*, 1979;*20*:137–145) reported that patients with PBC typically have a long and stable course, followed by an accelerated preterminal phase of hyperbilirubinemia, with a mean survival time of 1.4 years in patients with bilirubin of more than 10 mg/dL. The Mayo Clinic PBC survival model is based on patients' age, total serum bilirubin and serum albumin concentrations, prothrombin time, and severity of edema. These prognostic models have aided clinicians' decision-making process regarding optimal timing of LT, but they do not take into account fatigue, pruritus, or severity of bone disease in PBC. These complications must be taken into account separately when considering LT timing for patients with PBC. Nevertheless, these patients tend to have the highest levels of postoperative survival, with little risk of recurrent PBC after LT.

1.2.3. Primary Sclerosing Cholangitis (PSC)

PSC is a chronic cholestatic disease characterized by obliterative fibrosis of the bile ducts, leading to biliary cirrhosis and liver failure. Survival models have been developed based on such variables as age, serum bilirubin, histologic stage, and presence or absence of splenomegaly. The natural history of this disease includes recurrent cholangitis, progressive jaundice, or cholangiocarcinoma. The latter complication is an absolute contraindication for LT.

Besides offering potential therapeutic benefits, endoscopic retrograde cholangiopancreatography (ERCP) with biopsy and brushing of the biliary tract radicles is a common screening tool for cholangiocarcinoma. Early enthusiasm about CA 19-9 antigen and other serum tumor markers for cholangiocarcinoma has diminished following reports of poor sensitivity and specificity. Because of the risk of cholangiocarcinoma, patients with PSC should be referred early for LT.

1.2.4. Chronic Viral Hepatitis

Chronic viral hepatitis is one of the most common causes of end-stage liver disease, and this is reflected in the number of patients referred for LT. A better understanding of the mechanism of viral replication and of viral transmission has led to improved results with LT for patients with end-stage liver disease caused by viral hepatitis. Patients with *hepatitis B*-related liver disease (HBV) that are HBV-DNA negative can expect excellent survival after LT. Patients with *hepatitis D* virus (HDV) infection who are HBV-DNA negative can also expect an excellent survival rate. HBV-DNA-positive patients may patients may benefit from the addition of lamivudine to the prophylactic regimen both before and after LT. Lamivudine has proven to be effective in the treatment of both *de novo* and recurrent HBV infection after LT. However, viral resistance can develop.

Cirrhosis due to *hepatitis C* virus (HCV) infection is now the most common indication of LT in Western Europe and the United States. Although recurrent HCV infection was suspected to be the cause of posttransplant hepatitis in many of these patients, the actual incidence of reinfection was indeterminate until the development of polymerase chain reaction (PCR) tests for HCV in the early 1990s. It has become clear that graft reinfection is universal after LT for HCV. Recent data show that, despite universal reinfection of recipients, 5-year actual survival rate does not seem to be affected by the presence of HCV infection. However, liver biopsies may reveal an increased incidence of chronic hepatitis and cirrhosis in patients transplanted for HCV infection. An aggressive, acute cholestatic hepatitis can occur in 4–6% of patients transplanted for HCV within 6 months after LT. These patients inevitably will need retransplantation, but their overall post-LT prognosis is poor. Prognostic indicators have not been clearly delineated to determine which patients will do poorly after LT due to severe recurrence of HCV infection. One factor that is now widely accepted is an infected graft with HCV genotype 1. HCV+ donor to HCV+ recipient does not seem to be a predictive factor at this time. Post-LT therapy for HCV infection is investigational at this time, and trials with combination alpha-interferon and ribavirin are presently under way. However, a second LT for HCV-related allograft failure can be performed safely in patients, if performed before the onset of liver failure or other organ system failure.

1.2.5. Alcoholic Liver Disease

Alcohol abuse is the most common cause of liver disease, and the extent of application of LT to alcoholic liver disease remains controversial. Available evidence suggests that, among selected alcoholics, survival after LT up to 3 years is comparable to that of nonalcoholic patients. Cost analyses in North American transplant centers also suggest that resource utilization by alcoholic recipients is essentially the same as that by nonalcoholic recipients. A recent study from France (*Gut* 1999;*45*:421–426) concluded that LT can be successful in alcoholic cirrhosis, and that recidivism did not affect survival or compliance with immunosuppressive regimen. However, this area is still controversial. At present, most centers require 6 months of documented sobriety, psychosocial evaluation, completion of a rehabilitation program, and appropriate social support systems in place, before a candidate is accepted for LT.

1.2.6. Hepatic Malignancy

Hepatocellular carcinoma (HCC) is the most common primary liver malignancy. Surgical resection is an effective treatment for highly selected patients with HCC. Unfortunately, fewer than 30% of tumors are resectable. In selected patients with unresectable HCCs (single lesion ≤ 5 cm; or ≤ three lesions, each ≤ 3 cm), survival rates of 75% four years after LT have been reported (*Annals of Surgery*

1994;*219*:236–247). A recent study (*New England Journal of Medicine* 1996; *334*:693–699) comparing hepatic resection with LT in cirrhotic patients with HCC concluded that, in the face of severe organ shortage, HCC carcinoma developing in a well-compensated cirrhotic liver initially may be treated with hepatic resection, and LT should be applied selectively to patients with tumor recurrence and/or progressive liver failure. Long-term evaluation of adjuvant chemotherapy, including preoperative hepatic artery chemoembolization and postoperative chemotherapy, will further define the optimal approach.

1.3. UNCOMMON INDICATIONS FOR LIVER TRANSPLANTATION

LT has been successfully utilized as a therapeutic modality for numerous uncommon indications (Table 1.1). Because the products of hepatic synthesis permanently retain the metabolic specificity of the donor, patients with congenital enzyme deficiencies and other inborn errors of metabolism can be cured by LT. The cure afforded by LT is functional and phenotypic, not genetic.

Metabolic disorders considered for hepatic LT fall into two broad categories. Diseases not associated with any evidence of clinical or histologic hepatic injury include defects of the urea cycle, familial homozygous hypercholesterolemia, and primary hyperoxaluria. The other category consists of metabolic diseases dominated by hepatocyte injury, such as Wilson's disease, tyrosinemia, alpha-1-

TABLE 1.1. Uncommon Indications for Liver Transplantation

Metabolic and genetic deficiencies	Other
Alpha-1-antitrypsin deficiency	Amyloidosis
Familial hypercholesterolemia	Sarcoidosis
Wilson's disease	Budd–Chiari syndrome
Hemochromatosis	Veno-occlusive disease
Primary hyperoxaluria	Severe graft-versus-host disease
Protoporphyria	Hepatic adenoma
Crigler–Najjar syndrome	Polycystic liver disease
Urea cycle deficiencies	Alagille syndrome
Glycogen storage disease	Hepatic trauma
Lysosomal storage diseases	
Tyrosinemia	
Galactosemia	
Hemophilia A and B	
Cystic fibrosis	
Protein C, S deficiencies	

SOURCE: Rosen HR, Shackleton CR, Martin P. Indications for and timing of LT. *Medical Clinics of North America* 1996;*80*(5):1069–1102.

antitrypsin deficiency, and several types of glycogen storage disease. In contrast to other nonmetabolic liver diseases for which LT is performed, there is no risk of disease recurrence, and 5-year survival rates of 75% have been reported. Other systemic diseases for which LT has been performed include Alagille syndrome (arteriohepatic dysplasia), amyloidosis, sarcoidosis, cystic fibrosis, and severe polycystic disease.

1.4. CONTRAINDICATIONS TO LIVER TRANSPLANTATION

1.4.1. Absolute Contraindications

As LT has evolved, the list of absolute contraindications to LT has been refined, whereas the list of indications has expanded. Absolute contraindications (Table 1.2) make the outcome of LT unsatisfactory to the point that it should not be offered. Patients with *human immunodeficiency virus* (HIV) infection are generally excluded from consideration for LT. LT shortens the interval to development of acquired immunodeficiency syndrome (AIDS), and the majority of deaths post-LT in HIV-positive patients are related to complications of AIDS. *Extrahepatic malignancy* is also a contraindication for LT. Results of LT are so poor for patients with *cholangiocarcinoma* that most centers consider this malignancy an absolute contraindication.

Active alcohol or *illicit drug use* is an absolute contraindication to LT. At present, most centers require abstinence for 6 months before considering such patients for LT. Patients undergo psychosocial evaluation as part of their transplant

TABLE 1.2. Absolute Contraindications
to Liver Transplantation (LT)

HIV seropositivity
Extrahepatic malignancy
Cholangiocarcinoma
Hemangiosarcoma
Active sepsis
Active alcoholism or substance abuse
Fulminant hepatic failure with sustained ICP > 50mm Hg or CPP < 40mm Hg
Advanced cardiac or pulmonary disease
Inability to comply with immunosuppression protocol
Anatomic abnormalities precluding LT

CPP = cerebral perfusion pressure (mean arterial pressure minus ICP); HIV = human immunodeficiency virus; ICP = intracranial pressure
SOURCE: Rosen HR, Shackleton CR, Martin P. Indications for and timing of LT. *Medical Clinics of North America* 1996;*80*(5):1069–1102.

evaluation, primarily to identify adequate support systems to ensure that rehabilitation will be durable after discharge, and that compliance with medical care is maintained. Whether a patient should be excluded from LT because of advanced cardiac or pulmonary disease usually rests on the consensus of consulting specialists as well as members of the transplant team. *Coronary artery disease*, if mild or corrected by bypass surgery or angioplasty, is not a contraindication provided that left ventricular function is adequate. Advanced *chronic obstructive lung disease* or pulmonary fibrosis precludes LT. Following reports of improvement in arterial PaO_2 after LT, hepatopulmonary syndrome has become an indication rather than a contraindication.

It is important that the LT candidate be *free of active infection* before LT and onset of immunosuppression. This is particularly so because of the extensive upper abdominal surgery, multiple vascular and biliary anastomoses, prolonged period of anesthesia, and frequent need for extended ventilatory support in these patients. Serious chronic infectious diseases, such as osteomyelitis, chronic fungal disease, and abscesses, are significant contraindications to LT. The number of anatomic abnormalities that preclude LT has decreased with refinement of surgical techniques. Isolated portal vein thrombosis, previously an absolute contraindication, is now considered a relative contraindication.

1.4.2. Relative Contraindications

Conditions that may reduce the likelihood of survival after LT without being absolute contraindications are included in this group. It is often a combination of factors, rather than a single factor, that lead to the exclusion of a patient from LT. Furthermore, there is considerable variation from one transplant center to another regarding relative contraindications. The high recurrence rate and inferior survival rate associated with patients transplanted for *HBV-related liver disease* had led to the exclusion of HBV-related liver disease as an indication for LT at some centers. However, good results have been reported in patients who are HBV-DNA negative, have fulminant hepatic failure, or have HDV coinfection. These results have been achieved with the use of hepatitis B immune globulin (HBIg) therapy and with the recent introduction of lamivudine. Patients who are HBV-DNA positive remain at high risk for severe HBV recurrence after LT.

Patients *older than 65 years* are receiving LT with increasing frequency and are experiencing 1- and 3-year survival rates generally identical to those of their younger counterparts. They require vigorous evaluation pre-LT because of the increased risk of comorbid conditions, including cardiac and pulmonary disease, malignancy, and osteoporosis. Many centers believe that a well-motivated patient approaching age 70, who is physically active and mentally alert, may be a better candidate than an emaciated 50-year-old. The impact of *previous treated extra-*

hepatic malignancies on posttransplant outcome has been extrapolated from renal transplant literature. Low recurrence rates (0–10%) have been associated with renal tumors, lymphomas, testicular tumors, cervical tumors, and thyroid carcinomas. Intermediate recurrence rates (11–25%) occurred for carcinomas of the uterus, colon, prostate, and breast. High recurrence rates (≥25%) occurred for carcinomas of the bladder, sarcomas, malignant melanomas, nonmelanomatous skin cancers, and myelomas.

An important issue in LT candidates is *renal function*. In a multivariate analysis from Barcelona (*Hepatology* 1991;*18*:46A), renal function was shown to be the only independent prognostic variable for survival after LT for nonbiliary cirrhosis. Some centers consider severe hyponatremia a relative contraindication because of its association with central pontine myelinolysis. Severe malnutrition has been associated with longer hospital stay and poorer survival following LT.

Chapter **2**

Evaluation of Candidates for Liver Transplantation

Vivek Kaul, Kenneth D. Rothstein,
Santiago J. Munoz, Jorge Ortiz,
and Cosme Manzarbeitia

2.1. ORGAN MATCHING

The outcome of organ transplantation is an extremely complex phenomenon, being the result of an interaction between two different biological systems, those of the donor and the recipient. It is logical, therefore, that any discussion that attempts to describe the process of recipient evaluation must be initiated with a comprehensive assessment of donor and recipient variables. The benefits of "matching" donors to recipients are manifold. Stratifying prospective donor-recipient combinations provides valuable insight into the probable outcomes of individual patients and the analysis of factors that determine those outcomes. In addition, stratifying makes it possible to describe study populations stratified according to risk, and it allows for a uniform comparison of outcomes.

The United Network of Organ Sharing (UNOS) establishes policies regarding organ allocation based on a broad consensus and periodically amends these policies. The process of "matching" begins when a donor organ becomes available in the local area and is offered to patients on the waiting lists of the local transplant centers. In general, a donor is matched to the potential recipient on the basis of several factors (Table 2.1). Recipients are chosen primarily based on medical urgency and the time waiting on the list within each blood group. Using these criteria, if a donor organ cannot be matched locally to a recipient, then it

TABLE 2.1. Variables Involved in Organ Matching

ABO blood type	Identical > Compatible > Incompatible
Waiting time on list	Highest priority to candidate waiting longest
Degree of medical urgency	Status I > Status II A > Status II B > Status III
Body size	Determined by transplant surgeon

becomes available to patients outside the local area (e.g., regional). Conversely, local transplant centers also receive organs from distant areas if an acceptable match was not possible at the distant centers.

In addition to these variables, studies have attempted to identify potential donor and recipient factors that may have a bearing on graft and patient outcome and use this information for better matching. Several variables have been analyzed: Donor and recipient age, gender, body mass index (BMI), renal function, length of ICU (intensive care unit) stay, a history of cardiopulmonary resuscitation (CPR), and donor liver size have been studied with respect to graft and patient outcome. A study by Ploeg et al. (*Transplantation* 1993;*55*(4):807–813) indicated that reduced-size livers, older donor age, renal insufficiency before transplantation, and prolonged cold ischemic time were independently associated with a higher incidence of primary graft dysfunction. Several studies have shown the reduced graft survival seen in the subset of patients where a female donated a graft to a male recipient, but its clinical significance is questionable.

Unlike renal transplantation, liver transplantation (LT) is routinely performed successfully across major human leukocyte antigen (HLA) differences between donor and the recipient. In some studies, surprisingly, HLA matching has been shown to produce an unfavorable graft outcome.

2.2. CANDIDATE SELECTION

The overall goals of LT are to prolong life and to improve the quality of life. The selection of appropriate patients for LT to achieve these goals is a difficult task. Uniform minimal listing criteria that propose listing patients when their estimated survival with liver disease is less than that expected after LT were recently proposed and have generally been accepted. The salient features of this consensus statement are as follows:

- Agreement that only patients in immediate need of LT should be placed on the waiting list.
- Patients should not be placed in anticipation of some future need for such therapy.

- The most important non-disease-specific criterion for placement on the transplant waiting list was an estimated 90% or less chance of surviving 1 year (translates into a Child–Pugh–Turcotte [CPT] score of $\geq$ 7, Classes B and C) (Table 2.2).
- Cirrhotic patients who have experienced gastrointestinal bleeding caused by portal hypertension or a single episode of spontaneous bacterial peritonitis would meet the minimal criteria irrespective of their CPT score.
- Patients with fulminant hepatic failure, regardless of etiology of the onset of stage 2 hepatic encephalopathy, should be placed on the waiting list.
- A requirement for 6 months abstinence from alcohol before placement on the transplant waiting list was considered appropriate for most patients with alcoholic liver disease.
- The concept of "regional review boards" to review candidacy for LT in "exceptional" cases.

Allocation and distribution regulations of the UNOS have also recently undergone changes to balance the principles of utility (i.e., the overall benefits of LT to society) and justice (i.e., the needs of the individual patient).

In most transplant centers, a candidate selection committee comprises the transplant surgeon(s), hepatologist(s), psychiatrists, nurse coordinators, social workers and others, who determine the suitability and general priority for transplantation of potential candidates. Candidate selection is becoming an extremely challenging task with the need to continuously consider newer (and often, controversial) indications for transplantation, a virtually stagnant donor pool, and ever-

TABLE 2.2. Child–Pugh–Turcotte (CPT) Scoring System
to Assess Severity of Cirrhosis, as Adopted by UNOS

Parameter	Points		
	1	2	3
Albumin	> 3.5	2.8–3.5	< 2.8
Total bilirubin	< 2	2–3	> 3
Protime (↑ seconds) or INR[a]	1–3	4–6	> 6
Ascites	None	Controlled medically	Uncontrolled
Encephalopathy (grade)[b]	0	I–II	III–IV
For primary biliary cirrhosis, primary sclerosing cholangitis, and/or other cholestatic diseases: bilirubin (mg/dL)	< 4	4–10	> 10

*Note*CPT score 5–6: Child's Class A; CPT score 7–9: Child's Class B; CPT score 10–15: Child's Class C.
[a]The CPT Score includes either the prothrombin time (in seconds) or the International Normalized Ratio (INR).
[b]Encephalopathy is classified into four stages according the definition of Trey and Davidson.

TABLE 2.3. Criteria for Patient Selection for Liver Transplantation

I. Accepted indications for liver transplantation
   a. Advanced chronic liver disease
   b. Fulminant hepatic failure
   c. Metabolic liver disease
   d. Alcoholic liver disease[a]
   e. Hepatoma[b]
II. Controversial indications for liver transplantation
   a. HIV disease
   b. Older age (> 75 years)
III. No alternative form of therapy available
IV. No absolute contraindication to liver transplantation present[c]
V. Willingness and ability to accept liver transplantation and comply with follow-up care
VI. Ability to provide for the costs of liver transplantation and posttransplant care

[a]Documented abstinence and rehabilitation prior to listing for transplatation (usually a period of 6 months).
[b]Single lesion less than 5 m or up to three lesions, each < 2 cm in size.
[c]Uncontrolled systemic infection, current extrahepatic malignancy, AIDS, advanced cardiac/pulmonary disease, multisystem organ failure, and so on.

constricting health care budgets. The clinical, biochemical, psychosocial, and financial information regarding a patient referred for LT is first reviewed to determine if the patient meets the global selection criteria, highlighted in Table 2.3.

2.2.1. Workup of Candidates

The process of evaluating a patient in consideration for LT needs to address several key issues:

- What is the etiology of the liver disease?
- Does the patient meet minimal listing criterion for LT?
- Are there any contraindications to LT?
- Does the patient have any "severity of disease" indications for LT? (Table 2.4)
- Does the patient have any "quality-of-life" indications for LT? (Table 2.5)
- What is the psychosocial profile of the patient?
- What are the patient's social support systems?
- Is the patient willing and motivated to undergo a liver transplant?

A transplant hepatologist and surgeon, transplant nursing coordinator, social worker, and a financial counselor evaluate all patients referred for transplantation. If deemed appropriate, a psychiatric consultation is also requested. Once it is determined that the patient appears to be a suitable candidate for listing and

**TABLE 2.4. Severity of Disease
Indications for Liver Transplantation**

I. Chronic (hepatocellular) liver disease
   a. Hepatorenal syndrome
   b. Spontaneous bacterial peritonitis
   c. Serum albumin < 2.5
   d. Prothrombin time > 5.0 sec prolonged
   e. Serum bilirubin > 5.0 mg/dL
II. Cholestatic liver disease
   Serum bilirubin > 10 mg/dL

transplantation, laboratory, imaging, and other pertinent evaluations are carried out, as detailed in Table 2.6. Routine upper endoscopy is recommended to document the presence of gastroesophageal varices, portal gastropathy, and to rule out peptic ulcer disease and/or malignancy. Routine colonoscopic examination is not recommended but should be performed in patients with a history of unexplained weight loss and iron deficiency anemia. In patients with primary sclerosing cholangitis (PSC), for example, colonoscopy with biopsy of suspicious lesions is imperative to exclude high-grade dysplasia and/or malignancy. The individual patient's specific medical history and condition dictate any further investigations. For instance, patients with cholestatic liver disease should have a DEXA (dual energy X-ray absorptiometry) scan to exclude significant osteoporosis. These and any other special considerations that may impact posttransplant care are discussed in an ongoing fashion at the transplant selection committee meetings at most institutions.

**TABLE 2.5. Quality-of-Life Indicators
for Liver Transplantation**

I. Chronic liver disease
   a. Intractable ascites
   b. Spontaneous encephalopathy
   c. Variceal bleeding
   d. Incapacitating fatigue
II. Cholestatic liver disease
   a. Intractable pruritus
   b. Recurrent (> 2) episodes of biliary sepsis (cholangitis)
   c. Metabolic bone disease with fracture
   d. Xanthomatous neuropathy

TABLE 2.6. Evaluation of Potential Liver Transplant Recipients

Laboratory investigations

Complete blood count, Prothrombin time, partial thromboplastin time (PTT)
Chemistry (18) panel
Complete LFT (liver function tests) panel
Hepatitis A, B, and C serologies; HIV (Elisa)
Cytomeglovirus (CMV), Epstein–Barr virus (EBV), and herpes simplex virus (HSV) serologies
Autoimmune hepatitis markers (antinuclear antibody test (ANA), smooth muscle antibody (SMA),
    immunoglobulin profile, antimitochrondial antibody (AMA) if applicable)
Ceruloplasmin (age < 50 years), alpha-1-antitrypsin level
Ferritin, total iron-binding capacity (TIBC), and serum iron
Alpha-fetoprotein
Thyroid function tests
Urinalysis
Lipid profile
Drug and alcohol testing

Radiology

Chest X-ray
Hepatobiliary sonogram with Doppler study of portal system
CT of abdomen for liver volume estimation

Cardiovascular

Electrocardiogram (EKG)
Echocardiogram if patient > 40 years of age
Dobutamine echocardiogram/other stress tests if indicated

Pulmonary

ABG (arterial blood gases) test
Pulmonary function tests (PFTs), if indicated
Chest X-ray

Once the pretransplant evaluation is complete, the patients are generally assigned to one of the following four categories:

- Suitable and ready for transplant; to be listed for a donor organ.
- Suitable but not in immediate need of transplant; may be listed if he or she meets minimal listing criteria.
- Potentially reversible current/active contraindication; recategorization at later date after treatment and reevaluation.
- Absolute contraindication; transplant denied.

The more common indications and contraindications for LT are listed in Table 2.7.

TABLE 2.7. Common Indications and Contriandications for Liver Transplantation

Indication: Acute or chronic liver failure related to:	Contraindications
Chronic hepatitis (e.g., hepatitis B, hepatitis C, or autoimmune hepatitis)	Severe cardiopulmonary disease
Cholestatic disorders: primary biliary cirrhosis (PBC), primary sclerosing cholangitis (PSC), and extrahepatic biliary atresia	Uncontrolled systemic infection
	Current extrahepatic malignancy
	Severe psychiatric or neurological disorders
	Absence of viable splanchnic venous inflow system
Alcoholic liver disease	
Metabolic disease (e.g., Wilson's disease, hereditary hemochromatosis, alpha-1 antitrypsin deficiency, nonalcoholic steatohepatitis [NASH])	Lack of adequate financial/social support system
	HIV infection
Cryptogenic cirrhosis	Active alcoholism and/or illicit drug use
Fulminant hepatic failure of any cause	Any anatomic abnormality precluding liver transplantation
Hepatocellular carcinoma	
Polycystic liver disease	
Budd–Chiari syndrome and hepatic veno-occlusive disease	

2.2.2. Waiting Lists and Waiting Period

It is estimated that about 26,000 deaths occur annually from liver disease in the United States. Of these, about 1,300 occurred while waiting on the liver transplant list. Although the absolute number of donors has increased in the past years, the number of potential recipients listed for transplantation has overwhelmed it. Most recent UNOS data reveal that more than 13,000 patients are currently awaiting LT in the United States. With a relatively fixed donor pool of around 4,500 per year, this ever-increasing disparity between available donors and potential recipients has led to lengthening waiting periods and a burgeoning waiting list. The increased success and popularity of living donor liver transplantation (LDLT) programs across the country may help to correct this disparity to some extent. Although the overall death rate on the waiting list has decreased during the last decade, the death rate for the most urgent medical status patients (statuses 1 and 2A) remains very high and unacceptable.

In this context, the importance of the timing of referral for transplantation cannot be emphasized enough. Patients with cirrhosis should be referred for transplantation even before they develop evidence of synthetic dysfunction, experience their first major complication (ascites, spontaneous bacterial peritonitis, variceal bleed, etc.) or develop malnutrition. CPT Class A cirrhotics are best served by early referral to a transplant center, before they develop complications of cirrhosis. Lifestyle changes such as cessation of smoking and alcohol use can be introduced early in order to prevent cardiac and pulmonary complications. Patients can be entered into a screening program to monitor for development of hepatocellular carcinoma (hepatoma), with biannual ultrasounds and alpha-fetoprotein determinations. Early and timely referral for transplantation affords patients a reasonable and fair chance to outlive the long waiting period on the list.

2.3. OPTIMAL TIMING OF LIVER TRANSPLANTATION

Liver disease is the tenth leading cause of mortality in the United States. In 1997, it was responsible for 25,000 deaths. Since the advent of improved surgical techniques, intensive care monitoring, and immunosuppressive regimens, LT has evolved into a viable treatment modality for a large percentage of patients in liver failure. In 1999, 4,698 LTs were performed in this country. However, there are over 16,000 patients awaiting transplants, while the number of donors has essentially reached a plateau. The waiting list is estimated to increase by over 200% in the coming years. Currently, waiting-list mortality ranges between 15% and 30%. Although the use of extended donors, living related donation, and split liver modalities has marginally increased the donor pool, it is incumbent upon the transplant center to maximize scarce resources further by transplanting patients at the proper time. In addition, in order for LT to be successful, it should be offered to patients at a stage in which they are able to tolerate it from the physiological point of view. Before offering transplantation, we should give the native liver the opportunity to recover. It is important to transplant patients at a point in their illness when their likelihood of long-term survival without transplantation is low, yet they are physiologically sound enough to withstand a major operation and immunosuppression. This utilitarian approach is driven by medical as well as ethical and financial concerns. When properly timed, LT is medically and ethically rewarding, and financially prudent. This is the gist of the National Institutes of Health (NIH) consensus of 1983. The decision about when to proceed with LT centers around three particular clinical instances. These include the acute or fulminant hepatitis cases, the chronic or cirrhotic cases, and, finally, the issue of retransplantation.

In the late 1970s and early 1980s, the option of LT was thought of as a last-resort effort. Evolving throughout the 1980s, with the advent of cyclosporine, and into today, with even newer immunosuppressants, the frame of mind has dramatically changed. LT has evolved into a viable therapeutic option with good results. In the past, the patient was allowed to deteriorate to the point of being on life support in the ICU. Today, the option of LT should be thought of much earlier. The progression of the disease to the point of irreversible deterioration is so unpredictable, and sometimes so rapid, that transplantation should be thought of early in the course of liver disease. Proper timing of LT must take into account the etiology and natural history of the disease. Thus, different rules apply for acute or fulminant failure versus chronic liver failure. Additionally, retransplantation presents a number of ethical and physiological variables that must be addressed in order to serve the patient as well as the health care system properly.

2.3.1. Fulminant Hepatic Failure

Fulminant hepatic failure (FHF) is defined as acute liver failure complicated by encephalopathy in a patient with no prior history of liver disease. Two thousand patients per year develop acute liver failure in the United States. Irrespective of the cause, FHF causes sudden, massive necrosis of the liver in patients without any evidence of preexisting chronic liver disease. This term is not used for preexisting chronic liver disease or for acute Wilson's disease. Natural recovery happens in about 5–20% of cases. Before the era of cyclosporine, transplantation of the liver did not compare favorably with medical management alone. However, with today's overall survival rate of 88% for LT, FHF is an accepted indication for transplantation of the liver. The etiology of FHF remains largely undiagnosed, with up to 40% of cases being cryptogenic in origin. Other known etiologies include fulminant hepatitis A or B, toxic hepatitis due to acetaminophen or idiosyncratic drug reactions, and mushroom poisoning.

The decision to proceed with LT must be made expeditiously. The workup must be shortened and include essential blood work such as HIV and hepatic serology status, confirmation of diagnosis by repeated frequent liver function, and an ultrasound of the liver to determine patency of the portal vein and overall condition of the liver. The latter usually shows a shrunken liver with a patent portal vein. Successful determination of these parameters, as well as the etiology of FHF, will determine the final outcome with or without transplantation in this population. Poor prognostic signs include the existence of grade 3 or 4 encephalopathy, a severe coagulopathic state, and a rapid shrinkage of the liver as documented by ultrasound (or, whenever possible, computerized tomography [CT] scan). Other bad prognostic signs include metabolic acidosis, cardiovascular instability, or septicemia. It is important to monitor the progression of the brain dysfunction in FHF adequately to avoid transplantation of patients who otherwise are brain dead. Direct intracranial pressure monitoring and cerebral perfusion pressure have been utilized successfully. Transcranial Doppler ultrasound measuring cerebral perfusion pressure has also been used with variable results.

Mortality is therefore dependent on a number of factors, including etiology and proper timing of transplantation. A significant percentage of patients (35–50%) improve with intensive medical management alone. It is therefore important to identify those patients that will not respond to medical therapy but are still physiologically sound enough to tolerate transplantation. The King's College criteria (with some modifications) have emerged as the gold standard employed when evaluating the suitability of a patient for transplantation. Negative prognostic indicators for resolution of illness without transplantation (and therefore indications for transplant) include the following:

- Duration of jaundice greater than 7 days before the onset of encephalopathy.
- Factor V level < 20%, if younger than 30 years of age.
- Factor V level < 30%, if older than 30 years of age.
- Prothrombin time > 50 seconds.
- Total bilirubin > 300 μmol/L (17.6 mg%).
- pH < 7.3.
- Creatinine > 300 μmol/L (3.5 mg%).
- Grade III/IV coma.
- Less than 50% viable hepatocytes on liver biopsy.

These criteria vary slightly depending on the exact etiology of the acute liver failure. Generally, if a patient continues in the ICU with obvious signs of liver failure such as coagulopathy, altered mental status, hemodynamic compromise, and the aforementioned negative prognostic indicators, urgent workup should be initiated.

Unfortunately, patients lose their opportunity for transplant when contraindications arise in the end stages of their acute liver failure. Usually, these are infectious or neurological in nature. Pneumonias, urinary tract infections, and line sepsis are fairly common in this patient population. Active infection, whether from fungal or bacterial sources, is a contraindication to transplant. If the intracranial pressure (ICP) is greater than 50 mmHg, with a cerebral perfusion pressure of less than 40 mmHg (usually measured by placement of an intracranial monitoring device), or if signs of uncal herniation are seen clinically or on CT scan, the patient is generally not salvageable. Renal failure and acute respiratory distress syndrome (ARDS) are not contraindications. However, they present significant obstacles in the postoperative period.

The planning of transplantation in this particular population is problematic. If transplantation is performed across the board, many livers that would otherwise recover would be removed unnecessarily, subjecting patients to the risks of surgery and immunosuppression. However, waiting too long may expose the patient to septic and neurologic complications, as well as increase in overall mortality. In general, survival rate for transplantation for FHF ranges anywhere from 60% to 80%. This compares very favorably with the most advanced medical management techniques today. Thus, an early referral to a liver transplant center, the implementation of an aggressive evaluation protocol, and an early decision for liver replacement is the best algorithm for management of these patients. However, one should not underestimate aggressive medical management, as emphasized by King's College unit in London. The proper use of mannitol and hyperventilation to prevent brain swelling, as well as antibiotic prophylaxis, can bring many of these patients around without liver replacement. Other authors have successfully applied the use of prostaglandin E1 (PGE1) for cases of fulminant hepatic failure with varied success.

Certain causes of FHF, such as Wilson's disease or acute Budd–Chiari syndrome, should be treated with LT as soon as possible, because the prognosis with medical intervention alone is dismal. In the latter, a thorough evaluation for the presence of hypercoagulable states or malignancy should always be done.

2.3.2. Chronic Liver Disease

The vast majority of transplants are performed for patients with chronic liver disease. Indications may be infectious (e.g., hepatitis B and C), oncologic (e.g., hepatocellular carcinoma, metastatic neuroendocrine tumors), cholestatic (e.g., primary biliary cirrhosis, sclerosing cholangitis) or metabolic (e.g., amyloidosis, Wilson's disease). Although indications have expanded exponentially, the donor pool has remained relatively stable. In 1988, 36% of recipients waited more than 6 months for a graft. That number increased to 69% by 1997. In 1988, 22% of recipients spent more than 1 year waiting. By 1997, that number more than doubled to 48.3%. Therefore, scarce resources must be utilized optimally by maximizing the proper timing of transplantation.

All cirrhotics do not need transplantation. If well compensated (CPT Class A), their 1-year survival with optimal medical, radiologic (e.g., TIPS), and surgical (e.g., Sarfeh or Warren shunts) management exceeds that of transplant recipients. In cases of chronic liver disease, the patient should have an obvious indication for hepatic replacement, such as episodes of variceal bleeding, malnutrition, decrease in hepatic function, severe coagulopathy, spontaneous bacterial peritonitis, severe osteodystrophy, intractable pruritus, intractable ascites, severe encephalopathy, or any combination of the above. These patients are in the stage of hepatic decompensation. The expected 1-year survival of a decompensated cirrhotic is 10%. Each variceal bleed carries a 50% mortality rate. Patients with refractory ascites have a 50% chance of survival and a 25% chance of 1-year survival. Since decompensation can erode into the general well-being of the patient, he or she should still be physically strong enough both to participate in the recovery process and tolerate the procedure overall. Thus, the decision to proceed with transplantation includes close collaboration among the referring physician, the hepatologist at the transplant center, and the transplant team itself. The tip-of-the-iceberg effect of liver disease in certain patients, in which manifestations only typically happen in the late stages and in a sudden dramatic fashion, should alert referring physicians and the medical community at large about the importance of liver disease in the population. This can manifest as subtly as a progressive loss of intellectual capacity (subclinical encephalopathy) or lead to frequent hospitalizations for the aforementioned complications for liver disease. Growth and development problems are common in children with liver disease. These signs should alert the physician to refer for liver transplantation before development of the end-stage complications leading to death.

Recently developed, minimal listing criteria for transplantation includes a CPT score of greater than 7. However, different etiologies of liver failure are confounding variables when considering the optimal timing of transplantation. For patients with predominantly hepatocellular dysfunction, such as postnecrotic cirrhosis, hepatic function is lost well ahead of excretory function. In this group, the presentation is often with several complications, including coagulopathy, low albumin, malnutrition, ascites, and so on. In these cases, the clinician must take into account the following:

1. In alcoholic liver disease, abstinence should be maintained for a minimum of 6 months in order to lesson the risk of postoperative recidivism, to allow development of support systems and attendance of rehabilitation programs, and to allow the liver an opportunity to regenerate.
2. In cases of hepatocellular carcinoma, which frequently develops in cirrhotics, transplantation should be performed before the lesion metastasizes, becomes greater than 5 cm in size, or three in number.
3. In hepatitis B, transplantation should ideally be performed while there is no sign of active infection. Those patients transplanted with actively replicating hepatitis B DNA have a dismal prognosis. However, those transplanted with no signs of ongoing replication do extremely well with the addition of lamivudine and hepatitis B immune globulin both pre- and postoperatively.
4. Patients with Budd–Chiari syndrome who demonstrate cirrhosis or fibrosis on biopsy should be transplanted early, because their chances of extended survival without a new liver are small. However, prior to transplant, shunt options should be exhausted, especially in the acute situation.
5. Those patients with autoimmune hepatitis being treated with corticosteroids should be transplanted before the onset of extensive osteoporosis.

For patients with predominantly cholestatic disorders, a predominantly cholestatic picture with preservation of synthetic hepatic function till late in the course of the disease is the rule. The most studied model of disease staging and its relationship to posttransplantation outcome has been done in cholestatic diseases such as primary biliary cirrhosis, using the Mayo model. This complex evaluation takes into account age, bilirubin, albumin, prothrombin time, and edema. The life expectancy without transplantation can be predicted. This model allows preventing early transplantation in the patient who is still healthy and predicts the outcome with and without transplantation. However, this model is unique to cholestatic diseases, and few, if any, noncholestatic disease permit the application of this model in a more generalized fashion. As a general rule, the consensus is that transplantation should be done in the early stages of the disease, before the catastrophic complications of liver disease occur. Similarly, a PSC patient with the aforementioned negative prognostic indicators and recurrent cholangitis should be considered for transplantation. Because of the risk of cholangiocarcinoma in patients with PSC (about 10%), meticulous surveillance and expeditious workups should be performed.

Procrastination prior to referral to transplantation centers has resulted in undue mortalities both before and after transplantation. This should be avoided in those settings of chronic liver disease in which response to medical therapy is not well documented. In one study, 12% of candidates died while waiting, and most of these patients had been referred for transplantation while they were on ventilators, bleeding, coagulopathic, with hepatorenal syndrome, aspiration pneumonitis, subacute bacterial peritonitis, or a combination of these, as well as other added end-stage complications. In these cases, the outlook after transplantation is demonstrably degraded. One-year survival after liver transplant exceeds 85% in most centers. Patients who are transplanted before being placed on disability are more likely to return to work postoperatively. Those that receive livers while physiologically less sound have diminished survival rates. Therefore, consideration of transplantation should be an early, and not a late, decision. Sometimes rapid, unexpected deterioration occurs in patients with chronic liver failure. This is more frequently seen in those with parenchymal disorders. In these patients, extensive medical clearance is not possible. Those patients who develop progressive encephalopathy, hemodynamic instability, renal insufficiency, spur cell anemia, and coagulopathy unresponsive to the administration of clotting factors have an extremely poor survival rate and should be transplanted as soon as possible, before the development of medical contraindications or death.

Finally, an increasing number of diagnoses are being accepted for transplantation, such as polycystic kidney disease, neuroendocrine tumors of the liver, and inborn errors of metabolism. Expansions of several disease entities that affect the liver to the point of potential transplantation indications may further shrink the donor pool. Because of this, consideration of early listing of the potential hepatic transplant candidate is indicated.

Generally, it is important to optimize a candidate medically so that he or she can benefit most from transplantation. Electrolyte disturbances such as hyponatremia should be resolved outside of the operating room. Infectious issues (urinary infections, pneumonia, spontaneous bacterial peritonitis, tuberculosis, etc.) should be cleared before transplantation. Proper cardiopulmonary clearance is essential. Asthma and respiratory compromise secondary to ascites should be treated before surgery. Coronary artery disease should be addressed with proper screening and medical or surgical intervention when appropriate. In persons with a history of malignancy, meticulous workup should be performed to rule out recurrent disease. Generally, at least a 2-year waiting period after treatment of nonhepatic malignancy is recommended before proceeding with transplantation. Dietary habits, tobacco abuse, nutritional status, exercise tolerance, and psychosocial profiles should all be addressed prior to listing for transplantation.

2.3.3. Retransplantation: Whether or Not?

Before cyclosporine was available, retransplantation was a rare event. However, because of the increased survival rates and improved outcome, as well as the LT experience showing that patient survivals are consistently 10–15% higher than graft survivals, retransplantation is an option. A word of caution, however: It is obvious that these patients take priority in the current system by drawing organs from the pool of donors and removing them from those patients who have not yet received a transplant. Because the overall survival of patients with retransplanted livers is about 10% lower than those with primary grafts, the issue of whether this would be an acceptable algorithm still remains under much debate. Another reason why retransplantation becomes a less than desirable option to discourage is the fact that, if retransplantation were not widely available, most surgeons would opt not to use the so-called expanded donors. This would greatly limit the availability of current organ donors and have a bleak effect on transplantation today.

The overall retransplantation rate varies between 9% and 21%. The most common reasons for this procedure are chronic rejection (69%), primary graft nonfunction (36%), hepatic artery thrombosis (15%), acute rejection (22%), portal vein thrombosis, hyperacute rejection, bile duct necrosis, cholangitis, and recurrent diseases. In the tacrolimus era, retransplantation for rejection is less common than in previous time periods. Overall survival rates are approximately 20–30% inferior to those achieved in patients receiving primary transplants.

The timing of retransplantation in the immediate postoperative period is crucial because retransplants performed between days 1 and 4 after initial surgery are more successful than those performed between days 5 and 30. Data from the University of California at Los Angeles (UCLA) are similar, showing a significant decrease in survival in patients whose transplants were performed between 8 and 30 days postoperatively. Those patients with four organ system failures or the requirement of more than three transplants do not benefit from more grafts. Therefore, when a patient's graft shows poor function, manifested in continued acidosis, blood product requirement, hemodynamic instability, and encephalopathy, it is prudent to proceed to retransplant before infectious complication and multiple organ system failure ensues. If a biopsy shows more than 50% necrosis, a retransplant is indicated. Poor prognostic indicators are serum creatinine greater than 4, elevated serum bilirubin, age, need for mechanical ventilation, and greater than 12-hour donor ischemia time.

When transplant recipients show signs of graft failure later in their course, they should be listed when their CPT score is greater than 7, if no medical contraindications have arisen since their previous procedure. When performed electively, retransplantation can have results approaching those of primary transplantation. Anecdotal evidence shows that retransplantation for hepatitic C is best performed before the bilirubin is greater than 8 or renal failure ensues.

Because of the donor organ shortage and diminished survival associated with retransplantation, it is important to time the procedure appropriately. If contraindications have arisen, if the patient is not physiologically sound, and if the donor organ is not optimal, the likelihood of success is small. Therefore, the decision to intervene should be made prudently.

Chapter **3**

Management of the Patient Awaiting Liver Transplantation

Sammy Saab, Steven-Huy Han, and Paul Martin

3.1. INTRODUCTION

Protracted waiting times for patients awaiting orthotopic liver transplantation (OLT) place them at risk for developing potentially lethal complications of liver disease. In this chapter, we address the evaluation and management of these complications, including ascites, encephalopathy, pruritus, esophageal varices, and malnutrition.

3.2. ASCITES

Ascites remains one of the most difficult management problems in the OLT candidate (Fig. 3.1.). Paracentesis should be performed on initial presentation to confirm portal hypertension as the cause of ascites. As an initial treatment, salt restriction is efficacious in less than 20% of patients, thus necessitating diuretic use. Fluid restriction is recommended only if the serum sodium is less than 120 mEq/L. Rapid correction of hyponatremia should be avoided as it has been implicated in the pathogenesis of central pontine myelinolysis post-OLT.

Spironolactone is frequently used alone or in conjunction with furosemide. Dosages can be titrated up as necessary to achieve adequate natriuresis. Addition of hydrochlorothiazide may induce satisfactory diuresis in patients who continue to have significant ascites despite large doses of spironolactone and furosemide. Electrolytes, blood urea nitrogen, and serum creatinine should be monitored on

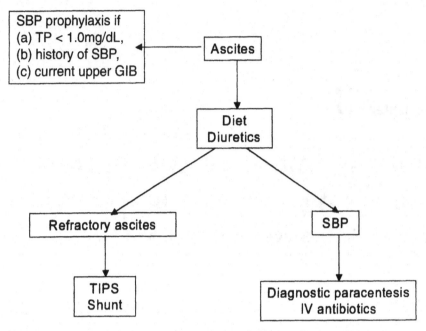

Figure 3.1. Algorithm for the management of ascites and its complications (SBP: spontaneous bacterial peritonitis; TP: total ascitic protein; GIB: gastrointestinal bleed; TIPS: transjugular intrahepatic portosystemic shunt; IV: intravenous). Typical doses for SBP prophylaxis are found in Table 3.2.

diuretic therapy. Diuretics should be discontinued if serum sodium falls below 120 mEq/L, or if the creatinine rises above 2 mg/dL. Hyponatremia in these circumstances reflects an excess of free water and should not be managed with hypertonic saline infusion. Alternative diuretic choices to spironolactone include amiloride or triamterene. In patients who are sulfa-allergic, ethacrynic acid may be used instead of furosemide.

3.2.1. Refractory Ascites

Refractory ascites (< 10% of cases) is defined as the inability to effectively diurese patients despite salt restriction and intensive diuretic treatment (spironolactone 400 mg/day and furosemide 160 mg/day). The limiting factor is usually the development of electrolyte abnormalities or renal insufficiency. It is important to exclude other causes of renal dysfunction, such as nonsteroidal anti-inflammatory drugs (NSAIDs). A 24-hour urine collection may be useful to confirm salt restriction and efficacy of diuretic therapy. Continued weight gain in a patient excreting greater than 78 mEq/L of urinary sodium in a 24-hour period suggests dietary noncompliance.

Repeat paracentesis may be performed every 2 or 3 weeks, though it is time-consuming, cumbersome, and may lead to excessive protein loss. The need for more frequent paracentesis suggests medical and/or dietary noncompliance. A transjugular intrahepatic portosystemic shunt (TIPS) may result in a significant decrease in ascites. However, TIPS may lead to compromised hepatic perfusion, with an increased risk of ischemic hepatocellular failure and intractable encephalopathy. Thus, TIPS is relatively contraindicated in Child–Pugh–Turcotte (CPT) Class C cirrhotic patients due to increased morbidity and mortality. Absolute and relative contraindications are listed in Table 3.1. Following TIPS regular surveillance for shunt stenosis with Doppler ultrasound is recommended. Most shunt occlusions can be revised radiographically.

Peritoneovenous shunting (LeVeen and Denver shunts) function by drawing ascitic fluid through a subcutaneous tube into the intrathoracic vascular space. Limitations include a high rate of shunt occlusion, disseminated intravascular coagulation, and increased perioperative mortality.

3.2.2. Spontaneous Bacterial Peritonitis (SBP): Treatment

SBP usually presents in cirrhotic patients as an unexplained clinical deterioration, as the classical signs of peritonitis, including fever, chills, and abdominal pain, may be absent. The mortality due to SBP remains high, reflecting the severity of the underlying liver disease. Paracentesis is diagnosed by finding an absolute neutrophil count (ANC) of greater than $250/mm^3$ in the ascitic fluid. Culture bottles should be promptly inoculated at the bedside to increase the yield. Empiric therapy should be directed at Gram-negative aerobic organisms and consist of a third-generation cephalosporin, such as cefotaxime, administered for 5 days. Antibiotic therapy should be tailored depending on the susceptibility profile of the infecting organism. Follow-up paracentesis is necessary if the patient does not appear to be responding to antibiotic therapy and to document a decrease

TABLE 3.1. Contraindications to Transjugular Intrahepatic Portosystemic Shunt

Relative	Absolute
Systemic sepsis	Intractable encephalopathy not precipitated by gastrointestinal bleeding
Hepatic neoplasms	Right-sided cardiac failure
Portal vein thrombosis	Severe hepatocellular failure
Polycystic liver disease	

in neutrophil count. Secondary peritonitis (i.e., due to a perforated viscus) should be suspected if the ascitic fluid Gram stain shows a polymicrobial flora, neutrophil count $> 10,000/mm^3$, brownish color, glucose < 50 mg/dL, lactic dehydrogenase (LDH) > 225 IU/L, or protein > 1 mg/dL.

3.2.3. Spontaneous Bacterial Peritonitis: Prophylaxis

Patients with a total ascitic protein of less than 1 g/dL, previous SBP, or recent upper gastrointestinal bleeding are at increased risk of developing spontaneous bacterial peritonitis and should receive prophylactic antibiotics (Table 3.2). Prophylactic antibiotic therapy is effective in reducing the incidence of SBP and is also cost-effective. Although there has been concern about the selection of resistant organisms with prophylactic antibiotic use, the clinical impact is unclear.

3.2.4. Hepatorenal Syndrome (HRS)

HRS occurs in approximately 10% of hospitalized cirrhotic patients. Diagnostic criteria for HRS are shown in Table 3.3. Currently, two distinct forms of hepatorenal syndrome are recognized. Type I HRS is defined as a rapid deterioration in renal function, with virtually all patients expiring within 10 weeks of onset. In contrast, type II HRS is insidious, with a life expectancy of several months. The major clinical consequence of HRS type II is the development of refractory ascites. Before a diagnosis of HRS can be established, other specific causes of renal dysfunction must be excluded, such as obstruction, volume depletion, glomerulonephritis, acute tubular necrosis, and drug-induced nephrotoxicity. A urinary catheter, renal ultrasound, and fluid challenge are useful in this setting. The recent use of nephrotoxic drugs (NSAIDs, aminoglycosides) is ruled out by history.

The treatment of HRS has been disappointing. Renal vasodilators (dopamine, prostaglandin, prostaglandin analogues), systemic vasocontrictors (norepineph-

TABLE 3.2. Prophylactic Antibiotics
against Spontaneous Bacterial Peritonitis

Antibiotic	Dosage (oral)
Ciprofloxacin	750 mg weekly
Norfloxacin	400 mg daily
Trimethoprim–sulfamethoxazole (double strength)	5 times per week

TABLE 3.3. Diagnostic Criteria for Hepatorenal Syndrome

Principal	Supporting
Chronic or acute liver disease with advanced hepatocellular failure and portal hypertension	Urine volume < 500 mL/day
	Urine sodium < 10 mEq/L
Serum creatinine (> 1.5 mg/dl or 24-hour creatinine clearance < 40 mL/min)	Unremarkable urine sediment
	Fractional excretion of sodium < 1%
Absence of shock, ongoing bacterial infection, use of nephrotoxic drugs	
No sustained improvement with diuretic withdrawal and expansion of plasma volume with 1.5 L isotonic saline	
No obstructive uropathy or parenchymal renal disease	

rine, octapressin), and antagonists of renal vasoconstriction (angiotensin II receptor antagonists, intrarenal phentolamine) have all been generally unsuccessful. Preliminary data suggest that the combination of volume expansion and systemic vasoconstrictors may help reverse HRS. In addition, a modified extracorporeal dialysis system may also improve HRS. TIPS may be useful, but its precise role remains to be defined for this indication.

3.3. ENCEPHALOPATHY

Between 30% and 70% of decompensated cirrhotics will have some degree of clinically obvious encephalopathy, which can range from subtle neurologic dysfunction to frank coma. The onset of encephalopathy requires a rigorous approach to identify and correct potential precipitants, as indicated in Figure 3.2 and Table 3.4. Serum electrolytes, blood urea nitrogen, and serum creatinine should be obtained, as well as a complete blood count to look for evidence of sepsis or blood loss. A urine toxicology test should be performed if there is clinical suspicion of illicit drug use, and ascites, if present, should be tapped to exclude SBP. Failure to respond to therapy within 48 hours should prompt a search for alternative mechanisms of intractable encephalopathy, such as portal vein thrombosis or occult hepatocellular carcinoma. Use of TIPS can lead to severe encephalopathy.

3.3.1. Treatment

Treatment revolves around identifying and correcting any precipitating factors. Patients can be given lactulose either orally, via nasogastric tube, or through

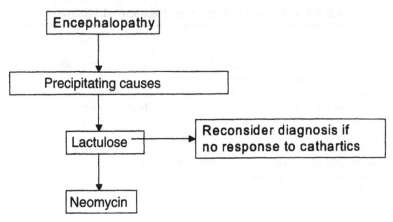

Figure 3.2. Algorithm for the management of hepatic encephalopathy (see Table 3.4 for list of common precipitating causes). Lactulose, 15 to 30 ml by mouth every 6 to 8 hours; neomycin, 1 to 3 g by mouth every 6 hours.

enemas (comatose or stuporous patients). The dose is titrated to achieve both two to four soft bowel movements daily and mental status improvement. If a patient continues to have encephalopathy despite correction of the precipitating event and adequate cathartics, neomycin may be added, though its potential for nephrotoxicity and ototoxicity can limit its use.

3.3.2. Benefits

Sufficient benefit has not been established for agents that stimulate metabolic ammonia fixation (ornithine-aspartate, sodium benzoate, and L-carnitine) in the

**TABLE 3.4. Common Precipitants
of Hepatic Encephalopathy**

Gastrointestinal bleeding
Constipation
Infection
Central nervous system depressive medications
Electrolyte disturbance
Portal vein thrombosis
Hepatocellular carcinoma
Transjugular intrahepatic portosystemic shunt

treatment of hepatic encephalopathy. Conflicting results in the use of branched-chain amino acids have led to skepticism about their use. The therapeutic role of flumazenil, a benzodiazepine antagonist in hepatic encephalopathy, remains to be defined.

3.4. PRURITUS

Most typically associated with cholestatic liver diseases, pruritus also occurs frequently in decompensated cirrhosis of other etiologies—most notably hepatitis C (HCV). Treatment strategies are summarized in Figure 3.3 and Table 3.5. Although cholestyramine is efficacious in about 90% of patients with pruritus, many patients find it unpalatable, and colestipol hydrochloride, another bile acid-binding resin, may be more acceptable. Other therapies include antihistamines, with dosing titrated to balance efficacy and sedative side effects, especially useful at night. The remaining 10% of patients with pruritus refractory to these therapies can usually be managed with rifampicin, with a significant reduction of pruritus. Because of the potential for bone marrow and hepatic toxicity, regular complete blood counts and liver tests are necessary. Ursodeoxycholic acid has its major

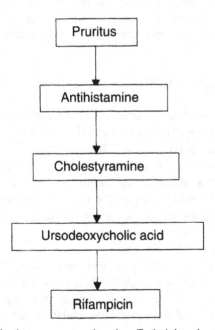

Figure 3.3. Algorithm for the management of pruritus. Typical drug doses are found in Table 3.5.

TABLE 3.5. Pharmacologic
Therapy for Pruritus

Drug	Daily dose[a]
Cholestyramine	4–16 g
Colestipol	5–30 g
Ursodeoxycholic acid	13–15 mg/kg
Antihistamine[b]	
Diphenhydramine	25–50 mg
Hydroxyzine	25–100 mg
Rifampicin	300–600 mg
Phenobarbital	2–5 mg/kg

[a]In divided doses.
[b]Commonly used antihistamines for pruritus.

indication in the treatment of cholestatic liver diseases, though it can alleviate pruritus in other forms of liver disease as well. Finally, opiate antagonists (naloxone, nalmefene, and naltrexone) have been used increasingly in the treatment of refractory pruritus, with significant decreases in daytime and nocturnal pruritus.

Malabsorption of fat-soluble vitamins often accompanies pruritus as a manifestation of cholestasis. As a result, prothrombin time and serum vitamin A and D levels should be monitored. Vitamin K should be used to correct a prolonged prothrombin time, and oral replacement of vitamins A and D provided.

3.5. ESOPHAGEAL VARICES

Bleeding from esophageal varices (EVB) is a major cause of mortality in patients with liver disease. The rate of variceal development is rapid, with 31% of cirrhotic patients having no EVB and 70% of cirrhotic patients with minimal EVB having large varices at 2 years. Mortality during the index EVB may reach as high as 50%. The risk of rebleeding within the first year is 70%. The initial management of EVB includes aggressive fluid resuscitation, administration of blood products to replace blood loss or correct coagulopathies as needed, and emergent endoscopic evaluation in an effort to control the bleeding source, as outlined in Figure 3.4 and Table 3.6.

EVB is a predisposing factor in the development of SBP and hepatic encephalopathy. Prophylactic antibiotics should be considered in all Childs B and C cirrhotics with EVB and ascites. Encephalopathy is a frequent consequence of the protein load from blood in the gastrointestinal (GI) tract after EVB and should be managed accordingly.

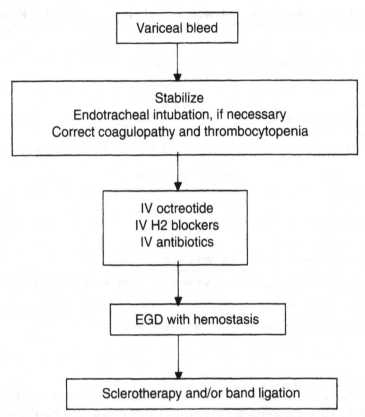

Figure 3.4. Algorithm in the evaluation and treatment of suspected esophageal variceal bleeding. Typical drug doses are found in Table 3.6 (IV: intravenous; EGD: esophagogastroduodenoscopy).

EVB classically presents with hematemesis and hemodynamic instability, though melena, hematochezia, or encephalopathy may be the initial manifestation. Close monitoring and prompt resuscitation is crucial, if necessary, initially with uncrossmatched O negative blood. A nasogastric tube should be inserted for gastric lavage. The sensitivity and specificity of the nasogastric aspirate for a diagnosis of EVB are 79% and 55%, respectively. If bleeding is likely to compromise the airway, endotracheal intubation is indicated. Patients should receive intravenous octreotide and H2-blockers. Alternatives to octreotide include vasopressin and nitroglycerin. Thrombocytopenia and coagulopathy should be corrected with fresh, frozen plasma and platelet infusion. After patients are hemodynamically stable, a prompt endoscopic evaluation of the upper GI tract should be performed. If esophageal varices are the documented source, endoscopic control should be attempted with rubber band ligation, sclerotherapy, or both.

TABLE 3.6. Pharmacologic Management of Upper Gastrointestinal Bleed[a]

Drug	Dose
H2-blockers (for potential nonportal hypertensive sources)	
Cimetidine	300 mg every 6 hours
Famotidine	20 mg every 12 hours
Ranitidine	50 mg every 8 hours
Splanchnic vasoconstrictors	
Vasopressin and	0.4 to 0.8 units per minute
Nitroglycerin[b]	40 μg per minute (titrate to systolic blood pressure > 100 mmHg)
Somatostatin	250 μg bolus, followed by 250 μg per hour
Octreotide	50 μg bolus, followed by 50 μg per hour
Vitamin K	10 mg once per day
Antibiotic	
Cefotaxime	2 g every 8 hours
Ciprofloxacin and	200 mg twice daily
Amoxicllin/clauvinillic acid	1 g/200 mg three times day

[a] All administered intravenously except vitamin K, which is given subcutaneously. Dose may need adjustment if serum creatinine is elevated.
[b] Alternative formulations include sublingual (0.6 mg every 30 min for 6 hr) and transdermal (10 mg every 24 hr).
[c] Ciprofloxacin and amoxicllin/clauvinillic acid can be administered orally.

Octreotide can be discontinued after several days if there is no evidence of recurrent EVB. Melena may take several days to clear. In the 5–10% of patients in whom endoscopic intervention is ineffective in controlling the bleeding, TIPS, balloon tamponade, or surgical shunts should be considered. Emergency surgical shunts have fallen out of favor because of substantial associated morbidity and mortality, as well as the availability of TIPS, though they are still indicated in CPT Class A patients.

Patients with cirrhosis should be screened for esophageal varices by upper endoscopy (Fig. 3.5). Evidence from meta-analysis suggests a potential role for propranolol in preventing/delaying the first EVB in patients with large varices. The dose of propranolol can be titrated to a resting pulse of less than 60 beats/minute or symptoms such as fatigue, dizziness, and depression. The combination of nitrates and nonselective beta-blockers is more effective than beta-blockers alone in preventing EVB, but few patients tolerate this therapy due to adverse effects. Prophylactic sclerotherapy has fallen out of favor, though emerging evidence suggests that esophageal variceal banding may play a role in preventing EVB. Similarly, secondary prevention using beta-blockers, sclerotherapy, or esophageal banding is efficacious in preventing recurrent EVB. Sclerotherapy is more effective than beta-blockade, and the addition of beta-blockade does not

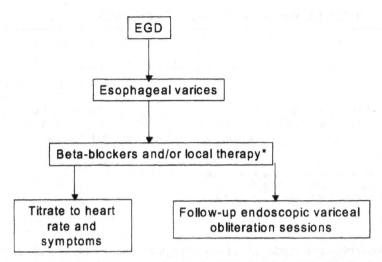

Figure 3.5. Algorithm for the management of suspected esophageal varices. Use of local endoscopic therapy requires availability of skilled endoscopists. Starting dose of propranolol (beta-blocker) is 20 mg by mouth twice daily. Goal heart rate should be 60 beats per minute. Adverse effects include fatigue and depressed mood (EGD: esophagogastroduodenoscopy).

appear to offer any advantages over sclerotherapy alone. There is a diminished risk of rebleeding with esophageal banding compared to sclerotherapy.

3.6. MALNUTRITION

Malnutrition is present in up to 60% of patients referred for orthotopic liver transplantation and carries a bad prognosis. There are several ways to assess nutritional status, as shown in Table 3.7. Besides the Subjective Global Assessment (SGA), which considers the presence of muscle wasting and subcutaneous

TABLE 3.7. Evaluation of Nutritional Status

Global subjective assessment	Laboratory studies
Subcutaneous fat loss	72-hour stool test for fat[a]
Muscle wasting	Vitamin levels, (A, D, and E[b])
	Prothrombin time

[a]If steatorrhea is suspected.
[b]Because vitamin E deficiency is rare, even in cholestatic liver disease, it should be checked only if neurologic deficits exist.

TABLE 3.8. Vitamin Supplementation in Cholestatic Liver Disease

Vitamin	Recommended replacement dose
A	5,000 to 20,000 IU daily
D	
25-hydroxy-vitamin D	50 to 100 μg daily[a,b]
1,25-dihydroxy-Vitamin D	0.05 to 0.2 μg/kg/day
E (κ-tocopherol, κ-tocopheryl acetate, κ-tocopheryl succinate	25 IU/kg daily
K	5 mg daily[c]

[a]Preferred form of vitamin D for supplementation.
[b]25-hydroxylated form of vitamin D_2.
[c]If prothrombin responds to trial of vitamin K.

fat loss, objective modalities of assessing nutritional status include anthropometric measures, bioelectrical impedance analysis, and creatinine height index. Objective measures do not substantially add more information to subjective assessment.

The approach to malnutrition includes evaluation of potential nonhepatic causes of malnutrition and addressing electrolyte and vitamin deficiencies. If malabsorption is suspected, a 72-hour stool collection for fat should be obtained. If stool fat is over 6 g/day, a trial of pancreatic enzyme supplementation is warranted. Patients with cholestatic liver disease are at an increased risk of fat and vitamin malabsorption. Vitamin A, D, and E levels and prothrombin time should be checked and corrected if necessary (Table 3.8). Patients should also consume at least 1,500 mg of calcium supplements daily. Patients with steatorrhea from chronic liver disease should reduce their total fat intake and consume a diet enriched in medium-chain triglycerides.

In the majority of patients, the cause of malnutrition is likely multifactorial. Inadequate diet, early satiety, and anorexia; altered substrate handling and metabolism; and depleted glucose reserve all contribute to malnutrition. Patients with

TABLE 3.9. Daily Diet Recommendation for Cirrhotic Patients Awaiting Orthotopic Liver Transplantation

Condition	Protein (g/kg body weight)	Total calories (kcal/kg body weight)
No encephalopathy	1.2 to 1.75	30–50
Encephalopathy		
Grade 1 or 2	0.5 to 1.2	25–40
Grade 3 or 4	0.5	25–40

malnutrition should not fast, should consume between 1.2 and 1.8 g/kg of protein daily, and have a total caloric intake of 30–50 kcal/kg/day (Table 3.9). Hepatic encephalopathy should not be considered a contraindication to a protein-containing diet. Nonanimal protein should be encouraged.

3.7. SUMMARY

Close monitoring of patients' overall status and interventions, such as prompt recognition of GI bleeding or SBP, is crucial to increase the likelihood of a patient surviving to benefit from OLT, the curative intervention for liver cirrhosis. Ameliorating some of the major causes of morbidity of cirrhosis, such as malnutrition, pruritus, and encephalopathy, improve the likelihood of a patient surviving until OLT.

Chapter **4**

Pretransplant Evaluation: Kidney and Pancreas
Jorge A. Ortiz, Cosme Manzarbeitia, and Radi Zaki

4.1. EVALUATION OF THE KIDNEY TRANSPLANT RECIPIENT

4.1.1. General Indications

The most common conditions that lead to chronic renal failure and end-stage renal disease (ESRD) requiring dialysis and evaluation for kidney transplantation (KT) are outlined in Table 4.1. Diabetes mellitus (DM) is the most common indication for renal transplantation. This is complicated by the fact that patients with DM on dialysis have a very high mortality. Some of these patients may be candidates for a combined kidney–pancreas transplant in its different modalities, as outlined later in this chapter. Chronic glomerulonephritis from various etiologies can lead to renal failure and ultimately necessitate KT. Polycystic kidney disease (PKD), an autosomal-dominant inherited disease, is most prevalent in Caucasians. Hypertensive nephropathy with nephrosclerosis, though widely prevalent, is more commonly seen in the African American population, due to the prevalence of hypertension in this group. Other causes of renal failure are less common and need individualized evaluation for KT.

4.1.2. Contraindications

Prior to recommending KT to any given patient, the diagnosis must be secured to avoid transplanting patients with reversible renal failure, such as those

TABLE 4.1. Indications for Kidney Transplantation

Etiology	% KT for this indication
Diabetic nephropathy	35
Glomerulonephritis with renal failure	30
Polycystic kidney disease	10
Hypertensive nephropathy with renal failure	10
Lupus nephropathy	3
Interstitial nephritis	3
Other	9

with acute tubular necrosis. Once the irreversibility of the process is clear, patients must be free of active infection (acute or chronic), active inflammatory glomerulonephritis (such as in active systemic lupus erythematosus [SLE]), active uncontrolled psychiatric disorder, and untreated malignancy). In addition, the patient must have a reasonable life expectancy after transplant and must be physiologically able to tolerate the transplant procedure. ESRD patients are prone to develop sequelae of arteriosclerosis and coronary artery disease (CAD), due in part to the higher incidence of hypertension and DM. The workup outlined here should also aim at excluding the consequences of other end-organ damage from these causes. High levels of sensitization to donor tissues also precludes transplantation due to a high incidence of hyperacute rejection and graft loss. This is further explained later in this chapter. Finally, patients must be compliant, without active addiction (alcohol and/or substance abuse), and highly motivated.

These contraindications may be absolute (e.g., intractable CAD with unstable angina), relative (e.g., hypertensive cardiomyopathy, which increases the operative risk but does not absolutely preclude transplant), or temporary (e.g., active pneumonia, which responds to therapy). All these circumstances must be properly weighed prior to considering a patient for KT.

4.1.3. Evaluation of Candidates

The evaluation and testing of the potential KT recipient follow the same general guidelines as those for the liver transplant recipient, as outlined previously, and are common also with the workup for combined kidney–pancreas transplantation. Patients must meet the previously outlined indications, be on (or about to go on) dialysis, and have irreversible ESRD. In addition, the progressive difficulty of obtaining adequate vascular access must be factored in the timing of transplantation for these individuals.

The workup starts with a detailed history and physical exam. Special emphasis is placed on the cause and evolution of the renal disease, time on dialysis, vascular access history and complications, urine production, presence of urologic issues that may complicate the future transplant (such as bladder neck obstruction or neurogenic bladder), medications, and, finally, review of systems to ascertain specific extrarenal organ system workup issues. A thorough psychosocial evaluation is undertaken at this time. Extensive laboratory, radiologic, and specialty testing then follow, as described later. When this is completed, the patient is presented for listing at a candidate selection multidisciplinary committee. If accepted, the patient is placed on the waiting list and financial clearance is established.

4.1.3.1. Blood Work

Laboratory studies include complete blood counts, full blood chemistry profiles, liver function tests, parathormone levels, and coagulation profiles. In addition, patients undergo serological testing for infectious diseases for viral (cytomegalovirus [CMV], herpes viruses, Epstein–Barr virus [EBV], hepatitis B and C [HBV, HCV], HIV) and bacterial (RPR for syphilis, purified protein derivative [PPD] for tuberculosis) diseases.

4.1.3.2. Tests, X-Rays, and Specialty Evaluation

Most patients undergo the following tests: chest X-ray, EKG, and abdominal ultrasound (size of kidneys, presence of hydronephrosis, gallbladder status). Urologic evaluation studies commonly performed include cystoscopy, urodynamic studies and a voiding cystourethrogram. Gastrointestinal evaluation includes upper and lower endoscopies as well as a hepatobiliary evaluation. Pulmonary assessment centers in the determination of clinically significant fluid overload, pleural effusions, or chronic pulmonary problems such as those caused by smoking habits.

Special emphasis is placed in the cardiovascular assessment. Patients undergo stress echocardiography, stress thallium scanning, and even coronary angiography to rule out CAD, cardiomyopathy, or endocarditis. Other important issues to consider include cardiac dysrhythmias and pericardial effusions. Finally, carotid duplex scanning and even peripheral angiography may be necessary to complete the evaluation in selected cases.

4.1.3.3. Specific Testing Based on Diagnosis

In cases of PKD, additional evaluation to rule out cerebral aneurysms is warranted. This can be done with either magnetic resonance angiography (MRA) or cerebral angiography. In certain disease such as SLE, the presence of a lupus anticoagulant must be ruled out preoperatively. A history of frequent, unexplained thrombosis of vascular access suggests a hypercoagulable state.

4.1.3.4. Tissue Typing and Organ Matching

Since the kidney allograft is very sensitive to antibody-mediated rejection, recipients undergo extensive immunologic studies. These assure proper matching of organs and minimize sensitization. Tests include ABO (A, B, AB, and O) blood typing, antibody screening, human leukocyte antigen (HLA) typing, panel reactive antibody percentage (PRA), and crossmatch (antibody reactivity) to donor tissue at the time of transplantation when a specific donor organ becomes available.

Organs are allocated based upon blood group matching, type of HLA matching, need for simultaneous kidney–pancreas transplant, time waiting, sensitization (PRA) status, recipient age and history of prior donation, and medical urgency. The allocation system is discussed in detail in another part of this manual.

4.1.4. Waiting Lists and Waiting Period

During the waiting period, both the nephrology team and the transplant team follows the ESRD patient. Scheduled serum samples are taken at regular intervals during dialysis visits to ascertain fluctuations of the PRA and crossmatch status. In general, waiting periods can be measured in years for these patients. During this time, dialysis allows for patient optimization, though progressive loss of vascular access can be a life-threatening factor, especially for diabetic patients. Also during this period, the patient may undergo surgical intervention aimed at optimizing the outcome of the future KT. These commonly include bilateral nephrectomy (e.g., for polycystic disease or chronically infected kidneys), cholecystectomy (for gallstones) and coronary artery bypass grafting (for CAD).

4.2. EVALUATION AND MODALITIES OF PANCREAS TRANSPLANTATION

4.2.1. Indications and Testing

Pancreas transplantation is established therapy for the treatment of Type 1 diabetes. As of 1998, over 11,000 transplants had been performed worldwide. *Indications* include the development of secondary diabetic complications such as renal insufficiency/failure, cardiovascular insufficiency, retinopathy, neuropathy, and life-threatening glucose unawareness. Over one third of type 1 diabetics develop ESRD. Ideally, the procedure is performed before the complications reach end stage. Pancreas transplant provides tight glucose control without insulin reactions and hypoglycemic episodes. However, it does this at a cost. Immunosuppression renders the recipient at risk for the development of certain cancers and many types of infection. For this reason, pancreas transplantation is only performed when the quality of life has become seriously impaired.

The *evaluation of candidates* follows a similar pattern to that of the kidney patient, with emphasis in the diabetic complications that can threaten successful transplantation. Consequently, great emphasis is placed on the cardiac and peripheral vascular workup. Cardiologic workup and clearance usually entails a peripheral vascular evaluation, chest X-rays, an EKG, a dobutamine stress echocardiogram, and frequently a coronary angiogram. Other common tests with other transplant recipients include serologic testing (i.e., CMV, HIV, HCV, etc.), HLA, blood group testing, complete blood count (CBC), and coagulation studies, to mention a few. Ophthalmologic, neurologic, and urologic workups are performed on a case-by-case basis (Table 4.2). Absolute contraindications include active infection, recent or current history of malignancy, positive crossmatch, and HIV infection. Relative contraindications include advanced age, obesity, and cardiovascular disease. Many centers consider that, in diabetics, severe end-stage retinopathy or limb amputations may contraindicate pancreas allografting.

4.2.2. Simultaneous Pancreas–Kidney Transplantation (SPK)

SPK has become an accepted therapy for the treatment of patients with insulin-dependent DM and renal failure or insufficiency (creatinine clearance < 70). The predialytic patient will benefit from the reduced costs, facilitated rehabilitation, and avoidance of complications associated with dialysis and uremia. Roughly 85% of pancreata are transplanted in this manner. Patient 1-year survival is over 90%, and graft 1-year survival is over 80%. The use of dual organs from scarce cadaver sources has caused some surgeons to perform live donor nephrec-

TABLE 4.2. Workup Testing of Kidney and Pancreas Transplant Recipients

System	Tests
Cardiovascular	EKG, stress echocardiogram, stress thallium imaging, coronary angiogram
Pulmonary	Chest X-ray, pulmonary functions tests
Gastrointestinal	Upper and lower endoscopies, gallbladder ultrasound
Urologic	Voiding cystourethrogram, urodynamic studies, renal ultrasound, cystoscopy
Peripheral vascular	Carotid duplex, peripheral vascular studies
Other	Pap smear, mammography, abdominal X-rays, CT of head, ophtalmologic evaluation, cerebral or other angiograms, dental clearance

tomy (usually laparoscopically) in conjunction with cadaver donor pancreas transplantation. The benefits include shorter wait-list time and increased long-term survival with live donor kidneys.

4.2.3. Pancreas after Kidney Transplantation (PAK)

If a Type 1 diabetic has already received a kidney from a live or cadaveric donor, a PAK transplant can be performed. A full 5% of pancreata are transplanted in this manner. The timing of the follow-up transplant does not seem to affect outcome. Assuming an acceptable organ has been procured and the recipient is healthy enough to withstand major surgery, the pancreas can be transplanted anytime after the kidney has been engrafted. Advantages of this technique include shorter wait-list times and the use of live donor kidneys, which yield greater kidney survival. Unfortunately, pancreas graft survival for PAK is significantly less than with SPK. Since results for pancreas transplantation are continually improving, this disparity is likely to decrease.

4.2.4. Pancreas Transplant Alone (PTA)

This technique has been traditionally reserved for the patient with life-threatening glucose unawareness, without secondary renal failure (i.e., with a creatinine clearance > 70). Roughly 5% of all pancreata are transplanted in this manner. Nowadays, more centers are performing pancreas transplants alone in order to correct glucose imbalance before the onset of secondary complications. Recent data state that diabetic lesions in native kidneys may regress after PTA. Unfortunately, the results have been inferior to transplants with kidneys and to transplants performed after prior kidney transplantation. Current 1-year graft survival rates for this modality stand at 52%. Most graft loss in the PTA group stems from rejection resulting from an inability to use serum creatinine as a marker for dual organ rejection. However, with newer immunosuppressants and the liberal use of pancreatic biopsy, some centers are reporting improved patient and graft survival.

4.3. TIMING OF KIDNEY AND PANCREAS TRANSPLANTATION

Due to the current availability of dialysis technology, an increasing number of patients with ESRD are surviving much longer now than they did in the past. Subsequently, a large portion of Medicare's budget is spent in providing dialysis and access for dialysis. Furthermore, dialysis has become an imperfect modality, fraught with problems of poor quality of life, demands of long periods of repeated exhausting therapy, loss of vascular access, complications of access surgery, and decreased sexual function. Transplantation, on the other hand, offers ESRD patients the opportunity to resume a normal lifestyle without the burden of dialysis and its associated complications. Economically, the cost of transplantation, medications, and follow-up is still less than the cost of the procedure for access and a dialysis regimen.

Transplantation, though the best therapeutic option for ESRD patients, is not always a viable one for several reasons. First, the number of cadaveric kidney transplantations has remained at a constant level despite the growing number of ESRD patients waiting on the list. This has resulted in the death of a growing number of patients waiting for a kidney transplant. Despite this, the demand continues increasingly to outstrip supply. Second, not every patient is a candidate for kidney transplantation. Cardiac disease, infectious processes, malignancies, chronic debilitating illnesses, and contraindications to general anesthesia all can preclude a patient's receiving a transplant. Third, once listed, the waiting time for a kidney is also excessive. Patients can wait on average 3 to 5 years on the kidney transplant list. Depending on the region in the country, this wait can be even longer. Finally, compliance issues can also preclude successful transplantation. Although compliance with dialysis regimens can be somewhat an indicator, accurately predicting patient compliance with medications at home and follow-up continues to be difficult.

ESRD patients have options. Once transplantation has been decided on and viability of the patient is determined, the option of *living related and living unrelated donors* can be presented to the patient and, possibly, to the patient's family. This alternative has multiple advantages over cadaveric kidney transplantation. First and foremost, the waiting period for transplantation can be eliminated. This means it is possible to transplant patients prior to their ever needing dialysis, thus avoiding the need for multiple access surgeries and the subsequent complications associated with the procedures. An added benefit of receiving a living related or living unrelated graft is that the donor is well known to the physician and can be thoroughly screened. The case can also be scheduled electively. Living related and living unrelated grafts have very low rates of acute tubular necrosis and graft nonfunction, and graft survival is superior to cadaveric graft survival. With the advent of laparoscopic donor nephrectomies and refinements of open techniques, the procedure is well tolerated, with low morbidity and mortality. Given these advantages, patients have realized this is the best option to avoid dialysis and resume their regular lifestyle. Transplant centers have also come to the conclusion that this option allows for the best possible result and provides a means for correcting the deficiencies associated with cadaveric kidney transplantation.

To allow the best possible outcome for ESRD, and allow for transplantation prior to initiating dialysis, proper *timing of referral* to the transplant center is crucial. The current dogma in management of ESRD is to begin the process of hemodialysis automatically. The change to a mentality of proper patient referral for transplantation rather than dialysis needs to be made. Proper monitoring of glomerular filtration rates (GFRs) in a nondiabetic patient with a GFR of 15 ml/min, and in a diabetic with 20 ml/min, is the key to correct timing of referrals for transplantation. This is the typical GFR at which patients are usually thought to require dialysis eventually and are referred to surgeons for access. Referral for transplantation at this time allows for appropriate preoperative workup and discussion for living related or living unrelated transplantation.

If transplantation is not feasible or available, the standard of care is *dialysis*. The two main modes of dialysis are hemodialysis and peritoneal dialysis. Indications for beginning dialysis include (1) GFR of 5–15 ml/min, (2) severe hyperkalemia, (3) metabolic acidosis refractory to medical therapy, (4) fluid overload, (5) uremic pericarditis, (6) neurological manifestations (e.g., lethargy, myoclonus, seizures), and (7) blood urea nitrogen (BUN) > 100 (not absolute—decreases morbidity and mortality). The timing of placement of access depends on the form of dialysis and type of access. *Peritoneal dialysis* via peritoneal dialysis catheter needs 2 weeks to mature prior to use. This form of dialysis, which requires an intact peritoneal membrane, has certain pros and cons. The major benefit to this access is independent lifestyle and shift of control of the therapy back to the patient. A major drawback to this form of dialysis is the inefficiency inherent in peritoneal dialysis. Persistent hyperkalemia and elevated BUN and creatinine levels leave patients uremic. Catheter infections can be frequent, depending on the hygienic practices of the patient, and may require removal of the catheter. Contraindications to peritoneal dialysis include multiple abdominal surgeries without an intact peritoneal membrane, abdominal aortic grafts, compliance issues of the patient, as well as the patient's lack of motivation.

In hemodialysis, the most common form of dialysis, there are many options when choosing forms of *access for hemodialysis*, such as temporary or permanent catheters, arteriovenous (AV) fistulas, AV grafts, and basilic vein interposition grafts. The superior form of access is an AV fistula, the varieties of which include the cephalic vein–radial artery fistula and upper-arm basilic vein–brachial artery fistula. The advantages to a fistula, once matured, are duration of patency lasting the life expectancy of a dialysis patient, with an extremely low incidence of thrombosis, as well as low infection rates. The disadvantages include time to mature (6–8 weeks) and requirement of a vein that is of sufficient diameter as well as superficial. The fistula also has the disadvantage of giving the patient a deformed appearance and requiring special training for the dialysis technician to access the fistula. With all these disadvantages, it is no surprise that only approximately 15% of all dialysis patients have AV fistulas.

AV grafts are the most widely utilized forms of access for hemodialysis. The material for the grafts is usually polytetrafluoroethylene (PTFE). Advantages to AV grafts include rapid time to maturity (2 weeks), easy access by dialysis technicians, and ease of placement. The disadvantages include low patency rates (6 months to 1 year), with frequent thrombosis, high rate of infection, higher incidence of steal syndrome, venous hypertension, and upper-extremity edema. The surgeon has many sites for placement of an AV graft. The preferred site is the nondominant forearm, followed by the nondominant upper arm, and then the dominant arm in similar fashion. AV grafts can also be placed in the lower-extremity, but this is not a preferred site due to patient comfort, higher incidence of lower extremity ischemia, and poor inflow due to secondary atherosclerosis. Therefore, these are usually sites of last resort.

The various forms of access for hemodialysis for a particular patient are dependent on multiple factors, such as life expectancy of the patient and comorbidities. Obesity or body habitus is a major determinant of the feasible form for a patient. The urgency of the need for dialysis also plays a role in the decision-making process. If a patient is in immediate need for hemodialysis, this might sway the surgeon to place an AV graft rather than a fistula. Patients with short-term life expectancy are better served with a temporary catheter (Permacath) placement than a formal AV access. Despite all of these factors that play a major role in determining form of access, the most important factor is still the size and status of the artery and vein. For example, the criteria for the size of a viable vein is 4 mm or larger for an AV fistula.

The timing of pancreas transplantation is covered in another chapter. Suffice to say that it is a function of whether the pancreas will be transplanted synchronously or metachronously to a kidney transplant, or whether it will be transplanted alone. Of course, the main indication for pancreas transplantation is intractable DM with associated ESRD.

Chapter **5**

Psychiatric and Social Workup of the Abdominal Organ Recipient

Kevin Hails

5.1. PSYCHOLOGICAL AND PSYCHIATRIC EVALUATION OF THE TRANSPLANT RECIPIENT

5.1.1. Screening

A transplant center should have some form of psychosocial screening for the transplant recipient. The screenings are an attempt to make certain that the potential recipient will have a good outcome, given that the transplanted organ is a scarce resource. Indeed, the screening process probably begins with the physicians who refer patients to a transplant center. They are probably screening out some patients before a referral to the transplant center is ever made. Obviously, little is known about the informal criteria used by these referring physicians, and there could be wide variation in criteria among these physicians.

The goal of the screening for the transplant psychiatrist is to identify any psychological risk so that treatment may occur. If treatment is not successful or cannot take place, then the patient may need to be rejected from the transplant program. The screening may also illuminate the needs of the patient and the family, so that planning for interventions or services can begin. It allows for the psychosocial team to establish a baseline of the mental functioning of the patient, so that postoperative behavior may better be understood. It also allows for continuity if services are needed postoperatively. The screening is usually done by a psychologist, a social worker, or a psychiatrist; or in some cases, a combination of the three. When the center has more than one discipline as part of the psychosocial screening process, there may be much overlap. This may allow the psychosocial team to confirm that there is consistency in the history as presented by the patient.

Olbrisch and Levenson (*Psychosomatics* 1995;*36*:236–243) posed several questions about the adequacy of the psychosocial screening process: (1) Are the psychosocial assessments able to predict postoperative outcome? (2) Are clinicians reliable in their evaluations of the transplant candidates? (3) Are the selections of candidates just and fair? (4) Can patients change their behaviors because of the experiences of terminal illness and transplantation when the change was difficult or not achievable before? The psychosocial team should work toward answering these important questions.

The transplant psychiatrist evaluates for any psychiatric disorders that may interfere with the transplant. He or she should also screen for self-destructive behaviors, compliance with medical treatment and the transplant workup itself, and any personality traits or disorders that may prove to be maladaptive. Psychotic disorders may make the patient unacceptable for a transplant if he or she becomes paranoid and noncompliant. However, a diagnosis of schizophrenia alone should not be an absolute contraindication to transplantation if the patient has a history of compliance with medication and is stable both psychiatrically and socially. Recurrent depressive disorders with multiple suicide attempts or failure to take care of one's needs would also be considered a contraindication. Even severe conditions such as borderline personality disorder could interfere with the ability of a patient to comply with the transplant protocol. Rapid shifts in mood, inability to sustain a positive relationship with the transplant team, and a narcissistic stance may render the borderline patient unacceptable. Severe eating disorders have also required rejection from the transplant program, secondary to the concern that the patient would induce vomiting and thus not be able to maintain a consistent blood level of immunosuppressants.

The psychosocial assessment must not attempt to discover the social worth of the patient. It is not uncommon for the patient to interpret the evaluation as such a vehicle. The patient should be reassured that this is not the case. Finally, the patient should be allowed to discuss his or her feelings about the transplant process. Candidates often have not had the opportunity to explore their concerns openly for fear they will be seen as inappropriate for a transplant. Indeed, the assessment can be therapeutic for the patient if the interviewer is supportive and empathetic.

It is important to verify the history presented by the patient with some other source, as the candidate may feel the need to "pass" the screening and may not give truthful answers.

Transplant centers need to be aware of the public debate about whether it is morally acceptable to treat alcoholic cirrhotics differently than other candidates. Most, if not all centers, believe that alcoholism is a medical diagnosis and that end-stage liver disease secondary to alcohol dependence, if in remission, should not prevent a patient's acceptance in a transplant program.

The evaluation of the *alcohol-dependent patient* is difficult. Although there is not universal agreement about the length of abstinence, most centers, including ours, believe that, with some exceptions, alcoholic patients should be abstinent for 6 months prior even to being considered for a transplant. In addition, any patient who has been abstinent for less than 3 years should be evaluated for the prognosis of maintaining abstinence. Ideally, both a transplant psychiatrist and an addictions specialist should do this. The psychiatrist should screen very carefully for any additional psychiatric diagnoses that would impact on the alcohol use of the patient. Some insurance companies require rehabilitation before they will consider paying for a liver transplant. The level of rehabilitation deemed necessary (inpatient, partial programs, and outpatient psychotherapy) is determined by the rehab specialist.

At our Center, a Beresford Alcoholism Prognosis Scale (Fig. 5.1) is also performed. This scale is intended for comparative purposes only. Its use presupposes that the clinician has made a diagnosis of alcohol dependence, as described in the third, revised edition of the *Diagnostic and Statistical Manual of Mental Disorders* (American Psychiatric Association. Washington DC: American Psychiatric Press, 1987), for any patient under study. The scoring system offers a method of quantifying clinical impressions for the purposes of statistical comparison. Neither the scale nor any parts thereof are used in isolation as a means of offering, or declining to offer, medical or surgical assistance. Additionally, most patients are required to sign a contract requiring that they remain abstinent before and after transplant, with random testing (Fig. 5.2.). It should be noted that patients who have a diagnosis of alcohol dependence have survival rates after transplant comparable to matched controls.

Drug dependence requires the same thorough evaluation by both a psychiatrist and an addictions specialist. Data are emerging to support the hypotheses that patients with polysubstance abuse are at higher risk to return to substance use than those who abuse only alcohol. Although current drug dependence is usually considered a contraindication to transplantation, methadone-dependent patients in a standing methadone maintenance program have been successfully transplanted several times in our program. The transplant program should be in close contact with the methadone program and look for patient compliance with the program's treatment plan and a stable relationship with the counselor. Dependence on prescription drugs poses a difficult challenge. The prognosis is improved if the patient maintains a good relationship with one physician, does not develop tolerance, and is on a minimum of medications.

ALCOHOLISM PROGNOSIS SCALE

Patient: _____

SSN: _____

1. Acceptance of alcoholism	YES	Patient and family	4 points
		Patient alone	3 points
		Family alone	2 points
	NO	Neither patient/family	1 point
2. Substitute activities:	YES		3 points
	NO		1 point
3. Behavioral consequences:	YES		3 points
	NO		1 point
4. Hope/self-esteem	YES		3 points
	NO		1 point
5. Social relationship:	YES		3 points
	NO		1 point
6. Social stability:	YES		3 points
	NO		1 point

Maximum Score—20 points
Minimum Score—5 points

TOTAL SCORE _____ Points

Figure 5.1. Beresford Alcoholism Prognosis Scale.

Transplant centers differ on the precise psychosocial and psychiatric criteria for inclusion into the program. Furthermore, there is variability among organ programs. Generally, renal programs are more relaxed than heart or liver transplant programs. The goal of the evaluation should not be solely to screen out candidates, but to propose a plan to allow inclusion into the program and to maximize the potential for those candidates that are already acceptable.

Many centers attempt to use psychological screening devices to assist in the selection of transplant candidates. However, Mori et al. (*Psychological Reports* 1999;*84*:114–116) question the validity of using the Minnesota Multiphasic Personality Inventory—2 (MMPI-2) or the Beck Depression Inventory for screening renal transplant candidates, because no significant differences were found between candidates seen as high and low risk based on other psychosocial criteria.

PATIENT CONTRACT

The following is a contractual agreement for the evaluation of a potential liver transplant recipient. This contract is supported by the Transplant Program and its team at _____ and will be ongoing from the initial evaluation. All potential liver transplant recipients with a diagnosis of alcoholic cirrhosis who have been abstinent for less than two years must go through a rehabilitation evaluation and adhere to their recommendations. The purpose of this Contract is to outline and document measurable guidelines and behaviors of the patient in recognizing inappropriate behavior and defining unacceptable candidates for transplantation.

Transplantation is a special opportunity for patients with end-stage liver disease to improve the quality of their lives. This program is dedicated to promoting and providing this option to all, in the restrictions of good self-care and responsibility. It is documented that transplant patients' noncompliance with medications, outpatient follow-up visits, and self- or substance abuse results in a higher degree of secondary complications and grafat failure. There is significant correlation with this to similar pretransplant behavior and compliance.

This contract will be used as deemed appropriate by the Transplant Team. It will be reviewed and explained to the patient, and the signature below will reflect understanding of expectations, purpose, and agreement to said terms.

The following conditions will result in failure to complete the contract and subsequently being deemed an inappropriate candidate for transplantation:

1. Resume ETOH consumption.
2. Positive drug screen for nonprescribed controlled substances (including cocaine) verified by random drug screen.

I agree to the terms and conditions of the above stated contract. I understand that my failure to comply with this contract may result in termination of my position as a potential transplant candidate. I also agree to allow any records from a rehabilitation specialist to be reviewed by the transplant team.

Reevaluation for failure to comply with the above contractual agreement will only be considered after a minimal time period of six months from the date of the failure.

Date: _____ Patient Signature: _____

MD Signature: _____

Transplant Coordinator: _____

Contract Date: _____

Figure 5.2. Institutional Patient–Transplant Team Contract.

Neuropsychological testing should be considered if there is concern that a transplant candidate suffers from a dementing process. Evaluation may be confounded by a subacute delirium, especially in the liver transplant candidate, but a careful history and serial evaluations can often clarify the situation.

Ethically, mental retardation should not be considered a contraindication to transplantation. Mentally retarded patients can do quite well following transplantation. A solid support system is a necessity. Obviously, a psychiatric evaluation for the decision-making capacity of the patient may be required and a substitute decision maker may need to be appointed.

5.1.2. Perioperative Period

The first issue in the psychiatric care of the transplant patient postoperatively is often the treatment of a change in mental status. A patient with an alerted state of consciousness, disorientation, hallucinations, and agitation or somnolence should be considered delirious. The first rule in treating a delirious patient is to correct the cause of the delirium. Electrolytes, liver function tests, complete blood count (CBC), magnesium, and blood gases should be part of the initial testing for a delirium. Immunosuppressants can cause delirium as well (to be discussed later). If the patient does not improve, then one should consider a central nervous system (CNS) infection because of the use of immunosuppressants or a vascular event. Haloperidol can usually be used safely in the delirious patient, as it does not depress respiration and has little effect on bowel motility, and rarely affects cardiac function. It can be given orally, intramuscularly, or intravenously, depending on the state of the patient. Cardiac function may be impacted with rapid intravenous (IV) infusion, as a few patients have developed torsades de pointes ventricular arrhythmias.

5.1.3. Postoperative Period

The postoperative period is a stressful one and patients often require a pharmacologic intervention for a preexisting or a new psychiatric disorder. The first issue for the psychiatrist is to determine whether symptoms represent a psychological response to stress or are secondary to medications or medical disorders. For example, the immunosuppressants have neuropsychiatric side effects associated with their use. Cyclosporine may commonly produce fine tremors, apathy, insomnia, anxiety, or agitation. Less common side effects are psychosis and delirium. Tacrolimus may produce tremulousness and sleep disturbances, especially if administered intravenously. OKT3 (a drug for acute organ rejection) may cause delirium. The use of corticosteroids may result in neuropsychiatric side effects. Females may be at higher risk. The side effects appear to be dose related and often involve mood changes. Haloperidol has been utilized to pretreat a patient who developed mania with steroids.

Patients in the postoperative period can develop psychiatric symptoms because of the stress of hospitalization, the disappointment of an outcome that is not what was expected, or a recurrence of an underlying psychiatric disorder. Patients who develop depressive or anxiety syndromes should be treated, if at all possible. However, patients may not require pharmacologic treatment simply for a brief period of distress. For example, a day or two of crying and distress may be perfectly normal and would not require an antidepressant. Decisions regarding the initiation of treatment should be made in conjunction with the psychiatric consultant. A major depressive disorder should not be diagnosed without the depressed mood being experienced most of the day, every day for 2 weeks. If the transplant patient requires psychotropic medication, caution should be exercised. Most psychotropic medications are metabolized in the liver, the exceptions being lithium and gabapentin. They are excreted by the kidney and should therefore be used with caution in the kidney transplant patient. There should be awareness about drug–drug interactions, since many psychotropic medications can inhibit the P450 enzymes. Strouse et al. (*Psychosomatics* 1996;37:23–30) found no significant interactions between fluoxetine and cyclosporine levels. Since sertraline also has no effect on the P450 3A4 enzymes, it would also be a good choice for a depressed patient.

The selective serotonin reuptake inhibitors (SSRIs) are generally safer choices than the older tricyclic medications, since the anticholinergic side effects may cause delirium or tachycardia. The tricyclics can cause blood pressure changes as well. The SSRIs do cause side effects such as gastrointestinal (GI) disturbances and headaches. Monoamine oxidase inhibitors (MAOIs) are best avoided because of the risk of hypertension. Ritalin can be another option, however. We have not found that it causes anorexia. Indeed, it may promote an increased appetite in some patients.

The psychiatrist and all members of the transplant team should ask patients what over-the-counter medications they are taking. For example, Saint John's wort has been associated with acute rejection because of an interaction with cyclosporine.

5.2. SOCIAL EVALUATION

The purpose of social workers in a liver transplant program is to assist in the identification and ongoing support of patients and families selected for liver transplantation. The intervention of the social worker can be better understood in phases.

5.2.1. Pretransplant Screening

The social worker, in conjunction with the financial coordinator, assists the patient and family in understanding the information regarding insurance resources (i.e., commercial, disability, Medicare/Medicaid, etc.) and private resources such as fund-raising. A written psychosocial history is obtained as part of the evaluation. The social worker interviews the patient and significant other(s) both individually and jointly. The psychosocial assessment comprises the following:

I. *Present living situation*
   A. Employment/education
   B. Nuclear and extended family composition
   C. Type of housing available/distance from the hospital
II. *Adjustment/compliance issues*
   A. Preillness responses to stress, usual coping mechanisms, and lifestyle
   B. History of psychiatric illness, drug or alcohol abuse, and smoking
   C. Understanding of the disease and its treatment
   D. Present emotional strengths and weaknesses
   E. Goals the patient has set posttransplantation/presence of strong desire to live
III. *Support system*
   A. Family relationships
      1. Stability of relationships, ability of support to make long-term commitment to providing emotional support to the patient both pre- and posttransplantation.
      2. Usual styles of communication, problem-solving patterns, role divisions
   B. Availability of other social supports: church, friends, extended family
   C. Insurance coverage
IV. *Potential problems/strengths*
   A. Highlight any area seen as problems or potential problems
   B. Highlight strengths

The social worker then presents the psychosocial evaluation at the interdisciplinary team meeting to determine patient candidacy for liver transplantation. The psychosocial selection criteria are as follows:

1. Patient demonstrates emotional stability and realistic perception of past and current illness.
2. Patient demonstrates a strong desire to live.
3. Patient has demonstrated ability to comply with medical treatment in the

past (i.e., taking medications appropriately, keeping appointments, carrying out treatment plans, compliance with rehabilitation treatment for addition, etc.).

4. A spouse, significant other, or family member is able and willing to make a long-term commitment for emotional/concrete support (to assist as needed with activities of daily living, etc.).
5. Adequate financial resources to meet the ongoing cost of medications.

5.2.2. Nontransplantation Candidates

In addition to the candidates, the social worker maintains periodic contact and provides follow-up linkage with community resources for those patients evaluated and deemed inappropriate for transplantation.

5.2.3. Waiting Phase

When the patient is accepted as a candidate for liver transplantation, the social worker maintains frequent contact with persons waiting at home and contacts hospitalized patients and their families three times weekly. The social worker provides ongoing counseling aimed at reducing anxiety during the waiting period and supporting the patient's coping mechanisms. Arrangements can also be made at this time for the patient and family to meet other transplant patients and their families.

5.2.4. Hospitalization Postsurgery

The social worker continues to follow the patient, spouse, and family for supportive counseling. Common areas of concern are as follows:

1. Reduced financial and social resources.
2. Anxiety regarding body image.
3. Concerns about roles in the family; concern about authority and self-esteem.
4. Family concerns related to adjustment to illness and hospitalization.
5. Anxiety regarding discharge.
6. Assistance regarding transportation for follow-up care.
7. Grief counseling and funeral arrangements.
8. Crisis intervention counseling as warranted for patient and family during course of treatment.

5.2.5. Discharge Planning

The social worker assists both patient and family in both the practical and emotional transfer from hospital to home and assists with any follow-up home care needs as warranted. After discharge, the social worker offers ongoing outpatient care by continuing to meet with the patients and families on a regular basis as part of outpatient clinic visits. Patient and social worker determine the frequency of meetings jointly. Support groups are usually held monthly for pre- and post-transplant patients and families. The group is led by a social worker and nurse. It is a combination education/support format, with suggestions for topics provided by patients and team members, and includes periodic guest speakers. Finally, the social worker also participates in interdisciplinary patient care meetings.

Chapter 6

The Role of the Transplant Coordinator

Laurel Lerner and M. Catherine Morrison

The needs of patients seeking transplants are diverse and complex, and best met by a multidisciplinary team. Cost constraints severely limit and challenge this dedicated group of health care providers to provide comprehensive, quality care. The transplant team usually consists of physicians, nurses, a social worker, and a financial counselor. Collaboration is essential for a thorough evaluation and comprehensive care of the patient.

The transplant coordinator is responsible for ensuring that all elements of evaluation and postoperative process are in place. The specific role of the transplant coordinator varies with each individual center. Most transplant coordinators take a central role and act as liaison among other team members. The goal is that the evaluation process be thorough and enlightening, and the postoperative period be uncomplicated. The role and responsibility of the transplant coordinator may also include reviewing and updating protocols, continuous program development, quality assessments, quality assurance, data collection, and research. This position requires an experienced, independent, mature individual with advanced assessment skills. Postoperatively, patient management becomes the transplant coordinator's primary responsibility.

Transplant coordinators at some centers share duties and care for patients from the initial evaluation through long-term clinic follow-up. Other centers choose to divide responsibilities into pre- and postoperative phases.

TABLE 6.1. Patient Medication Teaching Plan for Renal Transplantation

Definitions

A. Immunosuppression
B. Rejection

Immunosuppressive medication

A. Cyclosporine
   1. Formulations—Neoral, Gengraf, EON
   2. General instruction
      a. Take every 12 hours.
      b. Store bottle/gelcaps in cool, dark pplace. Available in 25 mg, 100 mg capsules, 100 mg/cc liquid.
      c. Take dose after laboratory blood sample taken.
      d. Do not remove gelcaps from foil packet until administration.
      e. Take liquid dose in glass container—rinse container and drink.
      f. May be taken with or without food.
   2. Side Effects
      a. Nephrotoxicity
      b. Hypertension
      c. Hair growth
      d. Hand tremors
      e. Gum hyperplasia
B. Prograf (Tacrolimus)
   1. Administration
      a. Take every 12 hours.
      b. Best taken on empty stomach.
      c. Take 2 hours apart from Cellcept (if on Cellcept).
      d. Available in 0.5 mg, 1 mg, 5 mg doses.
      e. Take after laboratory blood samples taken.
   2. Side Effects
      a. Nephrotoxicity
      b. Tremor
      c. Hair loss
      d. Increased blood sugar
C. Prednisone
   1. Dose and Taper
   2. Side Effects
      a. Moon face
      b. False hunger and weight gain
      c. Brittle bones
      d. Tissue sensitivity (bruises and ulcers)
      e. Slow wound healing
      f. Acne and mood swings
      g. Diabetes
      h. Sun sensitivity

TABLE 6.1. (Continued)

Immunosuppresive medication (cont.)

D. Cellcept (mycophenolate mofetil)
   1. Available in 250 mg and 500 mg tablets
   2. Take twice per day, 2 hours apart from Prograf (if on Prograf).
   3. Best taken on empty stomach.
   4. Side Effects
      a. Nausea, vomiting
      b. Diarrhea
      c. Leukopenia, thrombocytopenia
E. Imuran (Azathioprine)
   1. Available in 50 mg tablets
   2. Side Effects
      a. Leukopenia
      b. Hair loss
F. Rapamune (Sirolimus)
   1. Liquid 1 mg/ml
   2. Oral tablets 1 mg
   3. Side effects
      a. Hyperlipemia
      b. Leukopenia

6.1. PRETRANSPLANT COORDINATOR'S ROLE

Potential transplant candidates are referred to transplant centers most often by their nephrologist, gastroenterologist, or hepatologist. The evaluation process begins before the initial visit. The transplant coordinator obtains baseline information, including past medical history, past surgical history, etiology of disease, lab studies and psychosocial evaluation from the referring physician prior to meeting the potential recipient. Additional information is gathered at the first meeting and an evaluation plan is developed.

A bond is often formed at this initial meeting between the potential recipient and the coordinator. The transplant coordinator is in a unique position to become acquainted with the recipient. He or she becomes very familiar with the individual needs and preferences of the patient. Learning styles may be identified at this time.

Evaluation continues with a thorough history and physical. Specific psychological/medical problems that may interfere with a successful transplant outcome are identified at this time and will require further evaluation. Social support is vital to a good outcome and is assessed at this time. Family members, as well as potential donors, are encouraged to attend the initial visit at the transplant center.

Each center has a specific protocol for evaluation of candidacy. The transplant coordinator may assist the patient by scheduling appointments and assessing potential barriers to completing the evaluation. It is also the duty of the transplant coordinator to compile the results of the evaluation for presentation to the candidate selection committee.

Education remains the most challenging and core responsibility of the transplant coordinator. His or her ability to assess learning needs and learning styles, to formulate the learning plan, and evaluate results is the key to a successful transplant outcome. This educational process begins at the initial meeting and continues through the life of the transplant. The educational needs of the transplant recipient are overwhelming. Additional roadblocks to successful learning are low literacy skills, illiteracy, and physical handicaps (i.e., blindness). Patients often wait years for an organ and are likely to forget information presented at the initial meeting. A short hospital length of stay does not allow for a lengthy teaching plan. Information must be presented simply and continued at intervals postoperatively. The transplant coordinator teaches the recipient about the need for immunosuppression. The potential side effects and adverse reactions of anticipated medications are also reviewed.

Most transplant centers require 3 months of follow-up care before transferring patients to the referring physician for continued care. Some transplant centers continue lifelong follow-up. Patients often travel hours for their appointments, which is important to patients who must rely on others for transportation and child care arrangements, or who have financial constraints. Patients with drug- and alcohol-dependence problems are referred to the appropriate team member for rehabilitation prior to transplant.

The transplant coordinator notifies potential candidates when their names are placed on the waiting list for an organ. Candidates are also evaluated yearly by the transplant coordinator to assure ongoing candidacy. If the potential recipient has identified a living donor, compatibility is determined. If compatibility exists between the recipient and potential donor, the transplant coordinator then plans the donor evaluation.

Awareness and donation of organs have increased over the years but, unfortunately, have not kept up with the demand for organs. This is evidenced by the lengthy waiting time for organs. Transplant coordinators may also educate potential recipients, friends, and families about being tested for compatibility. When an organ is offered to the transplant team, it is usually the transplant coordinator who notifies the potential candidate. At this time, it is important to assess the patient for immediate contraindication to transplant (i.e., infection) and to notify the transplant physician.

6.2. POSTTRANSPLANT COORDINATOR'S ROLE

The roles of the pre- and posttransplant coordinators are similar in that education is a key component. The most important skill a patient can learn is independence. Teaching independence is challenging. The decreased length of stay post-

TABLE 6.2. General Guidelines for Transplant Recipients

Healthy living guidelines

A. Vaccines: Patients must always receive killed virus vaccines after transplantation.
1. Patient must avoid children who have received the live polio vaccine for up to 1 month; the child will secrete this virus through the GI tract. Do not come in contact with child's stools (i.e., changing diapers).
2. Examples of live or weakened vaccines:
    a. Smallpox
    b. Yellow fever
    c. Measles
    d. Mumps
    e. Rubella
    f. Oral polio
    g. Bacillus Calmette–Guerin (BCG)
    h. TY 21a typhoid
3. Examples of killed virus vaccines
    a. Flu
    b. Diphtheria–tetanus (booster only)
    c. Tuberculosis
    d. Pneumococcal
    e. Hepatitis B

Commonsense guidelines for patients

1. Wash hands frequently.
2. Avoid individuals who are ill.
3. Notify the transplant team if exposed to a communicable disease for the first time.
4. Watch for shingles and thrush.

A. Cancer
1. Immunosuppressive medications increase the risk of skin cancer. Skin should be shielded from the sun; patients should use sun block with a sun protection factor of 15 or greater and wear a hat and protective clothing if possible.
2. Female patients should receive a Papanicolaou smear annually.
3. Report any changes in skin, such as a change in size, shape, or color of a wart or mole.

B. Dentist
1. Patient must see a dentist every 6 months.
2. Antiobiotic coverage is needed for teeth cleaning, dental work, or any invasive procedure.

C. Activity
1. Walking is the best exercise initially.
2. Driving is permitted as soon as the patient's strength has returned to normal.

D. Sex
1. Use of a diaphragm or condom, or a combination, is the safest method of contraception for transplantation patients.
2. Pregnancy is strongly discouraged for 1 year after transplantation.

E. Smoking
1. This is strongly discouraged because of the increased risk of these patients for cancer and infection.

F. Returning to Work
1. Patients may return to work when they feel ready.
2. No heavy lifting (> 25 lbs) for at least 6 weeks after transplantation.

transplant poses a problem in readying the patient for discharge. Anxiety surrounding discharge also contributes to this challenge. Family members and significant others are enlisted as interim care providers until the patient gains independence.

The wealth of information needed before discharge is intimidating to many recipients and requires constant reinforcement. Patients with low literacy skills or physical disabilities present a unique challenge to the transplant coordinator. Evaluation of a patient's current knowledge base and his or her ability to learn is vital to the success of the teaching plan. Plans are individualized for these patients and, when necessary, help is enlisted from significant others. Creativity is encouraged to facilitate the learning process. Visual aides such as printed information, slides, and movies can be helpful. Patient management issues are especially evident in the posttransplant period. Compliance with follow-up visits and medication is stressed. If indicated, the reason for noncompliance is assessed and solutions are sought.

Before discharge, signs and symptoms of rejection, adverse reactions to medications, recommended routine screening, vaccine recommendation, exercise, and healthy living guidelines are reviewed. Tables 6.1 and 6.2 outline a formal, posttransplant medication teaching plan for a renal transplant recipient. Additional reinforcement or new teaching methods can be instituted to avoid complications. Outpatient clinic visits present an excellent opportunity to assess the patient for changing needs. As the patient recovers, new information may be introduced.

Communication with the referring physician is encouraged. Transplant centers provide a summary of the patient's course and recovery at time of transfer. Some providers are reluctant or inexperienced in providing postoperative transplant follow-up. Guidelines for patient management from the transplant center are helpful and can aide in the transition process for both patient and physician. This may include information on immunosuppressive medications, their side effects, and suggestions for laboratory values to be monitored. The transplant coordinator is available 24 hours per day at most transplant centers for physician and patient communication.

Transplant coordinators have a diverse and challenging responsibility to provide continuous care to the transplant patient. They are an integral part of the transplant team. Many patient issues that are not evident to other team members come to the transplant coordinator's attention. For this reason the transplant coordinator serves a vital role and link in the success of the transplant process.

Part **II**

Organ Procurement and Preservation

Chapter 7

Organ Donation and the Allocation System

Cosme Manzarbeitia

7.1. INTRODUCTION

7.1.1. NOTA, OPTN, and UNOS

Back in 1984, Congress passed the National Organ Transplant Act (NOTA) to establish a national system for allocation of organs in the United States. This act called for the formation of a national Organ Procurement and Transplantation Network (OPTN). The OPTN contract was subsequently awarded by the Health Care Finances Administration (NCFA) through the Department of Health and Human Services (DHHS) to the United Network for Organ Sharing (UNOS), an organization based in Richmond, Virginia. UNOS functions include organ allocation, transplantation, and scientific registry of transplant patients. All transplant centers, organ procurement organizations (OPOs), and tissue-typing laboratories have guidelines for membership in UNOS. This centralizes and standardizes the procurement and allocation of organs, assures standards of quality, and aims at maximizing organ usage and minimizing wastage. Within DHHS, the Division of Transplantation (DOT) controls both the scientific registry and the OPTN, and serves as vital link for OPO, promoting organ donation and transplantation through interactions with local, regional, and national organizations.

7.1.2. Death by Neurologic Criteria

Traditionally, death has been clinically defined as the cessation of all cardio-circulatory functions (i.e., cardiac arrest and death). Criteria for brain death were defined by the Ad Hoc Committee of the Harvard Medical School to examine the definition of brain death (*JAMA 205*,6, 1968, 337–340). Since then, all of the United States and many Western countries have endorsed this definition of death. Brain death is defined as the permanent and irreversible cessation of all cortical and brain stem function. This still allows other organ systems to maintain residual function (i.e., cardiocirculatory arrest is not needed to declare a person dead). This permits the procurement of organs while the major organ system functions (with the exception of the brain) are still preserved, thus giving an enormous boost to current organ donation and transplantation.

7.2. ORGAN PROCUREMENT ORGANIZATIONS (OPOS)

The OPOs coordinate all activities relating to organ donation and allocation at the local level. Their functions encompass education in organ donation, assistance to hospitals in the development of donation and procurement procedures, evaluation and management of donors, coordination of surgical retrieval and, finally, distribution of organs according to UNOS (OPTN) allocation rules. OPOs have evolved from a local hospital's efforts to involve independent, not-for-profit organizations. They abide by the OPTN regulations as administered by UNOS.

7.2.1. Donor Evaluation and Management

The evaluation of patients who have been identified as organ donors is performed on site by an OPO transplant coordinator. After proper donor identification, the coordinator usually confirms or facilitates the confirmatory tests for brain death and obtains consent for procurement from the family. Once this is secured, the goal of management is to determine the functional status of each organ system and to decide whether the different organs are suitable for donation and transplantation.

The goals of the management center around maintaining hemodynamic stability, appropriate oxygenation, biochemical homeostasis, and adequate organ perfusion. This usually represents a complete reversal of the management the patient had been receiving to the point of brain death. Thus, donors frequently need to be hydrated and to be given vasopressin to counteract diabetes insipidus, which is frequently seen after brain death. Though the detailed management of the brain dead organ donor is beyond the scope of this manual, suffice to say that management should be tailored to achieve an adequate balance to promote optimal preservation of function of as many transplantable organs as possible.

7.2.2. Administrative Coordination of Multiorgan, Long-Distance Retrieval

Once the donor is optimized, organs must be procured and allocated. The procurement techniques are described elsewhere in this manual. However, the procurement teams must go to the donor hospital to perform the recovery. The coordinator also aids with these arrangements, and, if an organ is procured locally but will be used at a distance, transportation arrangements are made, taking into account the maximum cold preservation time per specific organ. The on-site transplant coordinator, through the OPO, contacts the UNOS-based computer and runs a list of potential recipients for each specific organ that may be procured from the donor. The coordinator then contacts each center in that list to offer the organ, until each and every procurable and transplantable organ is properly matched with a prospective recipient. Once procured, organs are labeled, packaged, and sent to the transplant centers with the appropriate recipient, either along with the site-specific procurement team or shipped separately.

7.3. WAITING LISTS AND ORGAN ALLOCATION

Despite increased efforts by the transplant community to enhance organ donation rates, annual growth since 1995 has been flat, at an average rate of 1.5%. Meanwhile, waiting lists continue to grow rapidly at an annual rate of 15% per year. There is, therefore, great disparity between supply and demand. As of 1997, there were close to 60,000 patients on the waiting lists, with only about 13,000 organs procured in the same year (UNOS data, collected from *www.unos.org*).

Organs are generally allocated based on medical urgency and blood/tissue type matches. Kidneys and pancreas generally follow the same rules of allocation described below. Local lists are defined as those served by an OPO- or HCFA-designated service area. Regional lists follow the 11 regions adopted by UNOS; national lists cover the entire United States.

7.3.1. Allocation of Kidneys and Pancreas

For these organs, allocation and distribution are made first on a local, then regional, and finally national levels. The only exception is when a kidney has a six HLA–antigen match, in which case, national allocation and sharing is mandatory to improve outcomes. Allocation is made based on a point system that for its calculation takes into account the following factors: blood group, waiting time, type of HLA–antigen match, degree of sensitization (percentage of panel-reactive antibody), and age (pediatric vs. adult). Local patients with the highest points are allocated the organs in descending order; then, they are distributed regionally in descending point order, and finally nationally, in the same order.

7.3.2. Allocation of Livers

The subject of recent controversy, liver allocation schemes are currently in a state of flux. Currently, allocation takes into account degree of medical urgency, blood group, and time waiting, and also uses a point-based system for these factors. In addition, size is a consideration in preliminarily sorting potential recipients. Four statuses currently exist: 1, 2A, 2B, and 3. For status 1, organs are first shared regionally, then follow the local–regional–national scheme. Newer initiatives are being studied, such as the use of the Model for End-Stage Liver Disease score, a point system to predict mortality on the waiting list. Once validated, this may become the point system used to allocate livers in the future.

Chapter 8

Surgical Techniques for Liver Procurement

Sukru Emre and Cosme Manzarbeitia

8.1. WHOLE LIVER PROCUREMENT

There has been a gradual evolution of surgical techniques, from the meticulous *in vivo* dissection and removal of warm organs to the modern techniques and principles of the no-touch, en-block removal of *in situ*, core-cooled organs. For surgeons relatively inexperienced in donor hepatectomy and hemodynamically stable donors, it may be advisable to perform the hilar dissection prior to *in situ* cooling. Either approach is acceptable, so long as manipulation is kept to a minimum and rapid core cooling is instituted properly and promptly after cessation of circulation. The following is a list of *steps common to procurement of all abdominal solid organs*:

1. Prep and drape patient from the chin to midthighs.
2. An incision from the suprasternal notch to the pubis is made with electrocautery, and the sternum is split. Self-retaining retractors are placed on the sternum and the abdominal wall to allow full exposure.
3. The round ligament is divided and the falciform ligament and left triangular ligament of the liver are incised.
4. The left lobe of the liver is retracted with the surgeon's left hand and the crux of the diaphragm is incised with electrocautery. The supraceliac aorta is dissected and encircled for cross clamp later.
5. The inferior mesenteric vein (IMV) is exposed below the transverse mesocolon and cannulated to allow portal perfusion of the liver.

6. The infrarenal aorta at the level of the inferior mesenteric artery (IMA) is dissected and the IMA is ligated and divided. The aorta is then encircled at this level with umbilical tapes to allow for cannulation and aortic perfusion later.

7. The gallbladder is incised with electrocautery, and the gallbladder and biliary tree are flushed with saline solution to prevent autolysis during cold storage.

This is the full extent of preparation needed for liver and/or kidney graft removal. If a heart team is present, team members may then prepare their organ for removal. If no heart team is present or the team has completed its preliminary steps, heparin is given (20,000 to 30,000 U) and the distal aorta is ligated with umbilical tape. A large cannula is then placed in the distal aorta. Once the heart team has accomplished inflow occlusion of the superior vena cava, the aorta is clamped just proximal to the innominate artery by the cardiac team and simultaneously at the diaphragm, by the abdominal teams. The abdominal organs are then flushed with cold University of Wisconsin (UW, Viaspan®) solution via the IMV (portal) and aortic cannulas simultaneously. The vena cava is transected at the caval–atrial junction to allow free egress of blood and then perfusate. The cardiac team may then remove the organ; during this time, the liver is allowed to remain stationary and can be seen to blanch and become cool and asanguinous. Once the heart is removed and the hepatic surgeon is confident that the organ is well cooled and completely free of blood, formal hepatectomy is begun. The *steps for hepatectomy alone (pancreas not being procured) are as follows*:

1. The diaphragm is incised so that a small patch of diaphragm is removed with the liver, which encompasses the suprahepatic cava.

2. The right gastric arterial complex is identified, ligated, and divided close to the stomach.

3. The distal common bile duct is identified and transected.

4. Working in the groove between the upper border of the pancreas and the hepatic lymph nodes, the splenic artery, left gastric artery, and gastroduodenal arteries are identified, ligated proximately, and divided.

5. The portal vein is identified just superior to the upper border of the pancreas. Using blunt and sharp dissection, the surgeon traces it back to the confluence of the splenic and superior mesenteric veins. The portal vein perfusion is stopped, and the splenic vein and superior mesenteric vein are transected.

6. The distal portal vein is held superiorly and, with careful blunt and sharp dissection, the coronary vein and other small branches of the portal vein can be individually transected at a distance from the portal vein proper. Mobilizing the portal vein in this fashion, an anomalous right hepatic artery originating from the superior mesenteric artery can easily be identified and preserved.

7. The entire hepatic arterial supply can be mobilized to the base of the celiac artery, as there are no more vascular attachments. The celiac axis, along with the small patch of aorta, is removed.

8. The infrahepatic vena cava is identified and transected just above the origins of the renal veins. The remaining diaphragmatic attachments of the liver are divided sharply, and the right adrenal gland is bisected to assure protection of the upper pole of the right kidney. The liver is then removed and placed in a basin of ice (backtable).

9. Following hepatectomy, the kidneys may then be removed en-block.

Two common arterial anatomical variations must be recognized in the liver donor. First, an *accessory left hepatic artery*, originating from the left gastric artery in 10–15% of donors is recognized in the gastrohepatic ligament running transversely from the lesser curvature of the stomach to the umbilical fissure. Ligating and dividing the ascending and descending branches of the left gastric artery near the wall of the stomach may preserve this anomaly. This is most easily and commonly done prior to the dissection of the supraceliac aorta. The second most common variation, the presence of an *accessory right hepatic artery*, originates from the proximal superior mesenteric artery (SMA) in 15–20% of donors. This anomaly is easily identified once the portal vein is mobilized superiorly and is preserved by dissecting a long length of SMA distal to the anomalous artery. The entire SMA, together with the celiac artery, is removed on a common Carrel patch of aorta. Caution should be exercised while tailoring this Carrel patch to avoid damage to the renal arteries.

Backtable Preparation

A new portal infusion cannula is placed in the SMV and the liver is further perfused with 1 liter of UW solution via both the portal vein and hepatic artery. It is also advisable to flush the biliary tree with preservation solution as well. The liver is then packaged and transported to the recipient hospital for implantation. Once there, the hilar vessels are cleaned of superfluous tissue and the cava is cleaned of residual excess diaphragm, to allow for smooth anastomoses later. If any arterial reconstruction or lengthening of the vessels are needed, they are carried out at this time.

8.2. REDUCED-SIZE AND SPLIT-LIVER TRANSPLANTATION

If *reduced size liver transplantation* (RSLT) is contemplated, either a back-table left hepatectomy (for right-sided RSLT grafting) or a right hepatectomy (for left-sided RSLT grafting) is then performed. The vessels are thus kept with the portion intended for grafting, and during the parenchymal transection, the intra-parenchymal vessels are taken, with extra length toward the portion to be discarded. This maximizes hemostasis and allows for optimal hilar vessel length to facilitate anastomosis. After the nontransplant segment is removed, it is discarded, and the remaining graft is used as a RSLT graft. A variation of this technique would allow for preservation of reasonable length of the hilar vessels to both halves of the liver, allowing use of the two halves in two different recipients. In these instances, adequate length of hilar vessels may be problematic and interposition arterial or venous grafts, procured from the same donor, may become necessary prior to implantation. In this case the procedure is known as *split liver transplantation* (SLT). In SLT, two main procedures can be used:

- *SLT that produces left and right lobes.* In this case, the vena cava remains with the left lobe, as well as most of the caudate lobe. The right lobe takes the right hepatic vein for drainage. This is mostly used for SLT between two adults.
- *SLT that produces a right extended lobe and a left lateral segment* (Couinaud's segments 2 and 3, divided at the level of the umbilical fissure and drained by the left hepatic vein). This is used mostly for SLT between adults and children.

8.2.1. *In situ* Split-Liver Procurement

In these cases, the parenchymal dissection necessary to produce two transplantable, segmental liver grafts takes place in the donor hospital at the time of procurement. It usually involves dissection along the umbilical fissure and the edge of the falciform ligament to produce a right extended lobe and a left lateral segment. This is also mostly used for SLT between adults and children, as described earlier.

8.2.2. Living Donor Liver Procurement

Living donor liver transplantation (LDLT) has the advantage of availability of donor organs and may produce better long-term results than any other source of organs for pediatric or adult liver transplantation. This is a resource-intensive procedure, requiring the simultaneous use of a donor room and a recipient room, as well as two surgical teams.

In the pediatric population, most of the time, this involves *donation of a left lateral segment* (Couinaud's segments 2 and 3) from a relative. The resection starts with a careful dissection of the left hepatic artery within the hepatoduodenal ligament, with identification of the vital supply to the left median segment IV and the right lobe of the liver. Branches to the caudate lobe are sacrificed whenever necessary. The left lateral branch of the portal vein is isolated to obtain a single portal venous inflow to the graft. Dissection continues anteriorly along the round ligament separating the left lateral segment from the left median segment, along the medial edge of the round ligament.

The continuation of the round ligament between the posterior surface of the left lateral segment and the anterior surface of the caudate lobe is dissected to approach the left hepatic vein posteriorly. The left lateral segment is mobilized by the severing of the falciform ligament and the left triangular ligament, and the left hepatic vein is freed anteriorly. In the majority of cases, the left hepatic vein can be controlled extraparenchymatously. Finally, the bile duct is dissected and, after clear identification, encircled to be severed with scalpel at a late time. If necessary, the orifices of the median segment and the caudate lobe are sutured-ligated safely. The parenchymal dissection continues without vascular occlusion of either right or left lateral liver portions to avoid warm ischemia. The use of sharp and blunt dissection during the parenchymal dissection, with hemoclip application to larger vascular structures, is employed. Once full anatomical isolation is achieved, the hepatic artery, portal vein, and hepatic vein are clamped, severed, and taken to the backtable, where they are immediately flushed with UW solution through the portal vein and hepatic artery, and the bile duct is rinsed. If necessary, arterial and venous lengthening can be achieved using vascular interposition grafts from the donor-using saphenous vein.

Major limitations to *adult-to-adult LRLT* lie in the amount that can be safely removed from the living donor, which may be too small to function as a graft. Techniques using *full right lobes* (Couinaud's segments 5, 6, 7, and 8) appear very promising, though. The minimal need for donor tissue must be at least 1% of recipient weight. Ratios of < 0.7% are at high risk for the "small for size" phenomena leading to graft dysfunction. Intraoperatively, either the Cavitron Ultrasonic Aspirator (CUSA) and/or the Harmonic Scalpel is used almost exclusively in the donor procurements. The surgeon proceeds with the hilar dissection first, isolating the right branches of the portal vein and hepatic artery with vessel loops. Dissection and division between silk ties of the short hepatic veins draining the right hemicaudate are fundamental to identify clearly and isolate the right hepatic vein. Short hepatic veins larger than 5 mm in diameter are divided with the idea of reanastomosing them later in the recipient. The parenchymal dissection then proceeds along Cantlie's line till the bile duct is reached. Then it turns medially at a 30° angle to allow for proper procurement of the right hemicaudate and vessels to the right lobe. If the decision is made to heparinize the patient, heparin is used at doses of 3,000 to 5,000 units just prior to clamping the vessels, with minimal to no intraoperative bleeding. Once the parenchymal resection is complete, the portal vein is cut and bleeding from the specimen is allowed, and the hepatic artery follows suit. The dissection then proceeds to divide the right hepatic vein and the lobe is removed. Once removed, the lobe is weighed on the backtable and flushed with either UW or chilled lactated Ringer's solution, then taken to the recipient's room for implantation, which proceeds using the piggyback technique. Biliary reconstruction is done with either and end-to-end anastomosis over an internal stent if a single duct drains the donor right lobe. More commonly, however, two or more ducts necessitate that a Roux-en-Y anastomosis be fashioned.

8.2.3. Complications and Ethical Concerns of Living Donor Liver Procurement

The concern over ethical issues moderates enthusiasm for the use of living donors. The major ethical dilemma is justifying the exposure of an otherwise healthy donor to the risk of surgery and loss of all or part of a functioning organ to save the life of another person.

In patients with normal liver function and no general medical risk factors, the mortality associated with liver resection has been reported by several different centers to be as low as zero, but it has also been reported to be as high as 11%. The experience of Broelsch, Emond, and Heffron with almost 100 hepatectomies for benign disease revealed an estimated 1% risk of major morbidity and 5% minor morbidity (*Hepatology* 1994;*20*:49S–55S). These numbers support the fact that the liver has a high functional reliability. The vascular supply of the liver can be protected from trauma during liver resection, and regeneration of the remaining liver compensates for the loss of hepatic mass. Prior to the first living donor liver transplant at the University of Chicago in 1989, clinicians and ethicists deliberated for an entire year. This panel concluded that operative risk of surgical hepatectomy was low enough to allow parents or close relatives the option of donating a portion of their livers to children in end-stage liver disease (*Seminars in Liver Disease* 1995;*15*:165–172). A more general ethical issue is the question of whether the potential donor is free to make a voluntary decision. Family pressures or monetary compensation are examples of coercive factors that may affect a person's willingness to donate.

On the other hand, living organ donation has many advantages. Organs from living donors produce excellent outcomes, even with totally mismatched transplants. Donors are carefully screened and in excellent condition, and organ preservation times are short. Organs are sometimes of better quality than cadaveric grafts; 10% of cadaveric kidney grafts, for example, are damaged before removal. In addition, when a patient receives an organ from a person with whom he or she lives, the risk of noncompliance, and of losing a graft due to noncompliance drops, and the rate of rehabilitation rises. Another advantage of the living-related-donor approach is that once the donor is evaluated, transplantation can be performed promptly, while the patient has a relatively good prognosis. In contrast, if the disease progressed, deterioration in organ function would inevitably increase peri- and postoperatively, assuming the patient survived long enough to receive a transplant.

Living donor organs have enormous cost advantages over cadaveric transplants (i.e., the lack of procurement and shipping charges, the reduced complexity of laboratory tests, the lower cost implications of avoiding delayed early graft function and primary graft failure, and the consequences of less-maintenance immunosuppression). There is also a diminished financial burden to society as access to and equity of transplants are enhanced, with a reduction in the length of waiting lists for organs.

Studies also suggest that donating an organ may be associated with long-term psychological benefits to the donor. Donation is meaningful and altruistic. It promotes a closer feeling toward the recipient and a better life quality for the recipient and, in turn, the donor. Donors should be carefully informed, however, of the associated inconveniences, short-term risks of diagnostic procedures, and the pain and discomfort of surgery. There is also some financial risk for the donor, such as cost of travel to the transplant center and lost time and income during recovery. In addition, there are small psychological risks, such as minor depression in the immediate postoperative period. Depression is more likely to occur after graft failure, and donation can have an adverse effect on a marriage if the recipient is a spouse.

Critical protection might include providing a potential donor with all the information needed to make an informed decision. The transplant team should initiate rigorous psychological and psychiatric evaluations to ascertain the donor's ability to make voluntary choices. Mechanisms should be in place to monitor organ procurement and to minimize the influence of compensation. Transplant teams should reasonably establish the motives and reasons for living donor participation and make sure the choice is altruistic and not based on commerce.

Chapter **9**

Surgical Techniques for Kidney and Pancreas Procurement

Henkie P. Tan and Lloyd R. Ratner

9.1. CADAVERIC DONOR NEPHRECTOMY

Kidney procurement usually follows removal of the heart, lungs, liver, and pancreas. Many of the preliminary steps are common with multiorgan procurements, as described earlier. Once the abdominal viscera are flushed with the preservation solution, the kidney dissection is carried out in a bloodless field. A Cattell maneuver is performed to expose the aorta and inferior vena cava (IVC). The right lateral peritoneal reflection along the line of Toldt is incised, and the right colon is mobilized by retracting it superiorly and medially. Next, the small bowel mesentery is incised and swept up. The duodenum is mobilized (Kocher maneuver) and the pancreas is mobilized upward to expose the left renal vein, which is caudal to the celiac trunk and the superior mesenteric artery (SMA); these arteries are later ligated and then divided. The distal infrarenal aorta and IVC at the bifurcation are encircled with two umbilical tapes each (Fig. 9.1a).

The kidneys are dissected through Gerota's fascia, avoiding the renal hilum. To expose the left kidney, the left lateral peritoneal reflection of Toldt and splenic flexure are incised and the left mesocolon is divided. The ureters are transected distally as close to the bladder as possible. Periureteral areolar tissue containing the blood supply to the ureter is preserved. The ureters are retracted and freed to the level of the lower kidney pole. The IVC is divided just at the bifurcation. The

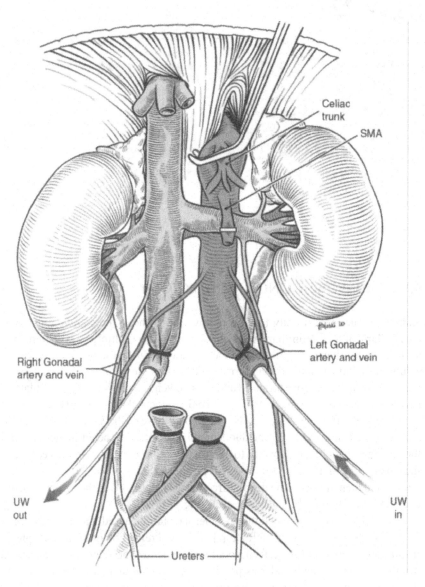

Figure 9.1a. Setup for procurement in cadaveric donor nephrectomy.

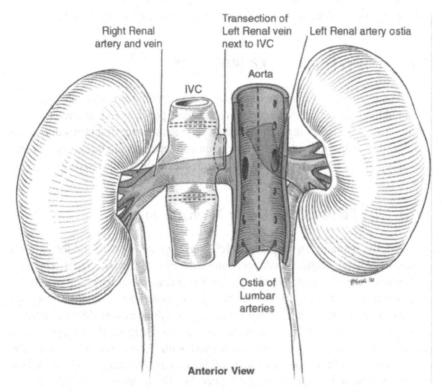

Figure 9.1b. Setup for procurement in cadaveric donor nephrectomy.

left renal vein is transected next to the IVC at the origin of the left renal vein to allow a panel graft of IVC to be created for extension of the right renal vein; the entire IVC stays with the right kidney. The aorta is then transected distally at the bifurcation and proximally, above the kidney. The kidneys, aorta, IVC, and ureters are retracted upward, and all tissues posterior are divided, while staying above the prevertebral fascia at the level of the paraspinal muscles. The aorta and IVC are incised vertically in the midline of the anterior wall to examine the orifices of the renal artery(ies) and vein(s) (Fig. 9.1b).

A Carrel's patch is created by dividing the posterior wall of the aorta vertically between the orifices of the renal arteries and the mirror-image orifices of the lumbar arteries. Care must be taken to identify multiple renal vessels, which are present in about 20–40% of cases. Sufficient perinephric fat should be excised in order to visualize the surface of the kidneys to rule out renal tumors and gross abnormalities. Before closing the abdomen, lymph nodes are taken from the small bowel mesentery or retroperitoneum, and a piece of spleen is removed for tissue type and crossmatch. The kidneys are packaged separately in plastic bags with University of Wisconsin (UW) solution and transported in ice coolers.

9.2. LIVING DONOR NEPHRECTOMY

The main principles in the living donor nephrectomy are adequate exposure, minimal hilar dissection, preservation of adequate perihilar and periureteral fat to ensure adequate blood supply to the ureter, and maintenance of diuresis during the operation. The left kidney, both in the open and laparoscopic techniques, is preferred because of the longer left renal vein and accessibility of the renal artery origin.

9.2.1. Traditional Open Donor Nephrectomy

Briefly, for a left nephrectomy, a left flank approach is used and the donor is placed in a lateral position, cushioned, and secured with adhesive tapes. The table is flexed to raise the flank. An oblique flank incision is made over the twelfth rib from the rectus anteriorly to the parasternal line posteriorly. The latissimus dorsi posteriorly and the external oblique anteriorly are divided. Dividing the internal oblique, transverse abdominis, and transversalis fascia enters the retroperitoneal space. The pleura are intimately associated with the peritoneum posteriorly, therefore care is taken to avoid a pneumothorax. Gerota's fascia is incised, and the kidney is dissected free from the perinephric fat. The ureter is identified medially near the gonadal vein and followed inferiorly, with preservation of the periureteric areolar tissue toward the common iliac artery bifurcation, where it is divided. Following the gonadal vein facilitates identification of the left renal vein. The renal vein is dissected to its junction with the vena cava, and the adrenal, gonadal, and lumbar veins are ligated and divided. The kidney is lifted upward and rotated anteriorly to dissect the renal artery to its aortic origin. At this point, mannitol and furosemide are given to promote adequate diuresis from the transected ureter. The donor is then heparinized. Once the urinary output from the kidney is assured, the renal artery is doubly ligated and the renal vein is oversewn with a running 4-0 Prolene suture. The heparin is reversed with protamine and the wound is closed. Chest X-ray is obtained to exclude the possibility of a pneumothorax. The patient is usually discharged from the hospital after return of intestinal function on the fifth postoperative day.

9.2.2. Laparoscopic Donor Nephrectomy

Despite the advantages of living donor renal transplantation, donors that undergo the open donor operation frequently are asked to forego approximately

10% of their annual income, experience significant pain, and pay out-of-pocket expenses for travel, housing, and child care. Prolonged recuperative time, pain, and cosmetic results are, therefore, disincentives to traditional live kidney donation. Thus, the laparoscopic living donor nephrectomy was specifically designed to address the significant financial and logistical disincentives to open live kidney donation.

9.2.2.1. Preoperative Evaluation

Preoperative evaluation ensures that the potential donor is left with normal renal function after unilateral donor nephrectomy. All potential donors undergo extensive medical and psychological evaluation in accordance with guidelines published by the American Society of Transplantation. A very useful test for preoperative radiologic evaluation of living donors is dual-phase spiral computerized tomography (CT) scan with three-dimensional angiography.

9.2.2.2. Surgical Technique

The operative procedure for the laparoscopic live donor nephrectomy has been described previously in detail. A left nephrectomy is described here. After induction of general anesthesia and preoperative antibiotic, a Foley catheter and an orogastric tube are placed. The patient is placed in the modified flank position with the torso in a 45° lateral decubitus position and secured to the table. The hips are rolled slightly posterior to allow exposure to the lower abdominal midline. The arms are flexed and placed at chest level with appropriate axillary and lower extremity padding. The table is then flexed. Pneumoperitoneum up to 15 mmHg is established using a Veress needle in the subcostal region. Three transperitoneal laparoscopic ports are placed, as depicted in Figure 9.2a. The first 10/12-mm port is placed lateral to the rectus muscle, halfway between the umbilicus and iliac crest using an optical trocar (Visiport RPF optical trocar, U.S. Surgical Corp., Norwalk, CT). The second 10/12-mm port is placed at the umbilicus and a 5-mm port in the midline between the umbilicus and xiphoid, both under direct vision. The umbilical port is used primarily as a camera port throughout the dissection. A 30° lens is used for visualization during the procedure. The AESOP 1000 robotic arm is employed (Computer Motion Inc., Goleta, CA) to hold and direct the laparoscope during the procedure. During the operation, the patient's fluid volume is kept expanded to maintain renal blood flow and good urine output. Patients are routinely given in excess of 5–7 L crystalloid intravenously, in addition to diuretics.

After pneumoperitoneum is achieved, laparoscopic Debakey forceps (in the 5-mm port) and scissors (in the lateral port) are used to incise the lateral peritoneal reflection of Toldt. The colon is then reflected medially, beginning at the splenic flexure, to the level of the sigmoid colon by incising the phrenocolic ligaments

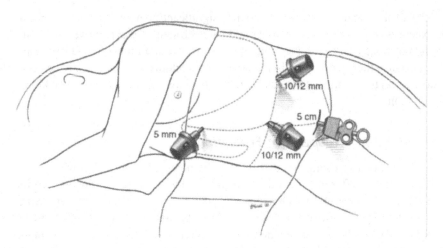

Figure 9.2a. Laparoscopic donor left nephrectomy patient position. The three port placements (10/12 mm, 5 mm, 10/12 mm) are noted. The fourth port is placed in the midline through a short Pfannenstiel 5 cm in length.

completely. Extreme care is used to avoid thermal injury to intra-abdominal viscera when using the electrocautery. The lienorenal and lienocolic ligaments at the inferior border of the spleen are divided, allowing the spleen to be retracted superiorly. The posterior attachments to the spleen may also need to be divided to mobilize the spleen and splenic flexure medially. The renocolic ligaments are divided and Gerota's fascia exposed. The upper pole of the kidney is then completely freed within Gerota's fascia. Dissection is facilitated with gentle elevation of the upper pole with a blunt retractor (Fig. 9.2b).

Care is used to avoid dissection at the hilum. The left renal vein is freed from its adventitial attachments, and the gonadal, adrenal, and, usually, one lumbar vein may be identified, doubly clipped on both sides and divided sharply (Fig. 9.2c). Maximal vascular exposure should be achieved by completely dissecting the renal artery to its proximal origin at the aorta. To prevent vasospasm, the renal artery is frequently bathed with a topical solution of papaverine (30 mg/ml). At this point, the patient is given 12.5 g of mannitol and 40 mg of furosemide intravenously. The lateral, posterior, and inferior attachments to the kidneys are left intact. This three-point fixation limits the mobility of the kidney and prevents torsion on its vascular pedicle. Attention is then focused on the urethral dissection inferiorly. The gonadal vein is again identified and a plane is created medially toward the sidewall. This dissection proceeds inferiorly down to whether the ureter crosses the iliac vessels. The gonadal vessels are then clipped doubly on both sides and then transected at the level of the pelvis, where they cross anterior to the ureter. The

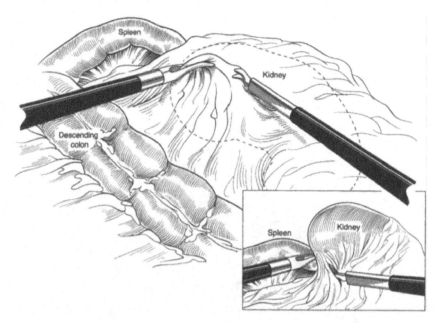

Figure 9.2b. Division of the colorenal ligament and exposure of Gerota's fascia. Inset: The upper pole of the left kidney is freed and elevated.

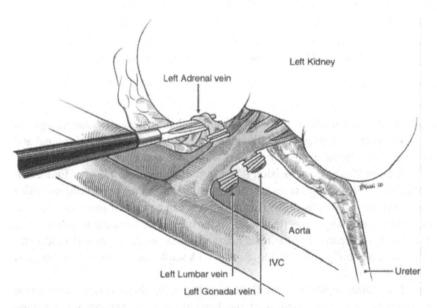

Figure 9.2c. The left renal vein is exposed and the gonadal, lumbar. and adrenal veins are doubly ligated and divided.

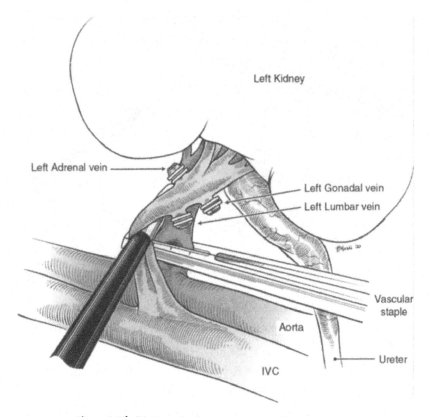

Figure 9.2d. Division of left renal artery and vein sequentially.

ureter is then transected at the level of the left iliac vessels after double ligation with a 10-mm clip applier. The remaining inferior, lateral, and posterior renal and ureteral attachments are finally divided with sharp and blunt dissections.

A 5-cm Pfannenstiel incision is made at this time, and a 15-mm Endocatch bag (U.S. Surgical Corp.) is inserted while maintaining pneumoperitoneum with a circumferential suture ligature. This instrument can be used to assist in retraction of the colon medially if inserted earlier in the operation. The patient is then given 3,000 units of heparin, and the renal artery and vein are then transected individually and sequentially with an endovascular GIA stapler (Autosuture, U.S. Surgical Corp.) (Fig. 9.2d).

The kidney is placed in the Endocatch bag under direct laparoscopic vision by grasping the perirenal adipose tissue. Once secured, the peritoneum is opened and the kidney is gently delivered. The donor kidney is then quickly flushed with

500 ml iced preservation solution after its delivery. Protamine sulfate (30 mg) is given intravenously and the abdominal fascia are closed with interrupted No. 1 absorbable sutures. The renal bed followed by the trocar sites is inspected for hemostasis. The fascia of the 12-mm trocar ports are closed with No. 1 absorbable suture. For right-sided laparoscopic donor nephrectomy, the operation is technically more difficult, because the liver must be retracted cephalad to allow dissection of the upper pole. The midline port between the xiphoid and umbilicus is placed more superiorly. A blunt instrument is required to retract the undersurface of the liver to the right sidewall. Exposure of the short right renal vein at the level of the vena cava is accomplished after the duodenum is kocherized. To remove the kidney, a 6- to 8-cm right-upper-quadrant transverse incision is made. This incision is made when the entire kidney has been mobilized and the ureter divided. The renal artery is ligated proximally and divided, and the right renal vein is divided after placement of a Satinsky clamp across the IVC to allow maximal length of the renal vessel. The vena cava can be closed with 4-0 Prolene or the VCS clip applier (U.S. Surgical Corp.).

9.2.2.3. Results

Patients who undergo laparoscopic live donor nephrectomy, compared to the open flank approach, resume full activities (2.2 ± 0.8 weeks vs. 4.2 ± 2.4 weeks) and return to employment sooner (3.9 ± 1.8 weeks vs. 6.4 ± 3.1 weeks). In the subset of patients that perform physically demanding jobs, the laparoscopic cohort reported that patients felt able to return to work significantly sooner than the open group (3.8 ± 2.7 weeks vs. 8.0 ± 4.0 weeks). The length of hospitalization was also significantly shorter for the patients that underwent the laparoscopic operation (2.9 ± 1.0 days vs. 5.5 ± 1.2 days, $p < .001$). In addition, the perioperative analgesic requirements, complications, readmission rates, and estimated blood loss were significantly lower in the laparoscopic group.

9.2.3. Complications and Ethics of Living Donor Kidney Procurement

In the Johns Hopkins laparoscopic donor nephrectomy experience, donor morbidity has been acceptable. In the first 171 living donor nephrectomies, complications related to the operation were seen in 25 patients (14.6%). These included 3 (1.8%) open conversions, 1 (0.6%) reoperation, 6 (3.5%) blood transfusions, 5 (2.9%) wound infections, 7 (4.1%) transient thigh paresthesias, 1 (0.6%) incisional hernia, 1 (0.6%) pneumonia, and 1 (0.6%) bowel injury. This is comparable to the open procedure. Waples et al. (*Urology* 1995;*45*:207–209) reported an overall complication rate of 17% in a retrospective 20-year review of 681 open donor nephrectomy patients. In a recent study by Johnson et al. (*Transplantation* 1997;*64*:1124–1128), an overall complication rate of 8.2% was noted in 871 open donor nephrectomies. Of note, complications that are not uncommon with the open donor operation, such as pneumothorax, incisional hernia, and chronic wound pain or discomfort, are virtually nonexistent with the laparoscopic operation. Of more importance, to our knowledge, there has been no associated laparoscopic donor nephrectomy mortality in any of centers currently performing laparoscopic live donor nephrectomies.

Of comparable importance to the safety of the donor is that the recipient outcome, graft survival, and cost are at least comparable. No significant differences were observed in patient or graft survival; incidence of technical complications (ureteral or vascular); incidence, timing, or severity of rejection episodes; need for dialysis; hospital stay; or long-term creatinine clearance between recipients of open versus laparoscopically procured kidneys. As with complications in the laparoscopic donor nephrectomy, the recipient ureteral and vascular complications generally occurred early and appeared to be a function of the learning curve. Of timely interest in the current cost-conscious health care environment, there was no overall difference in total hospital charges between these two groups either. In addition, the complication rates and readmission rates were lower for the laparoscopic compared to the open procedures.

9.3. CADAVERIC DONOR PANCREATECTOMY

9.3.1. Pancreas without Liver Procurement

Pancreas without liver procurement usually includes bilateral kidney procurement. The main technical details include the preservation of the gastroduodenal artery. The proper hepatic artery, distal to the gastroduodenal artery, and the left gastric artery are ligated and divided. A cuff of aorta, including the celiac axis and superior mesenteric artery in continuity, is excised with the pancreaticoduodenal graft. The portal vein is transected high in the hilum of the liver to preserve the length of the portal vein.

Briefly, a midline incision from the suprasternal notch to the symphysis pubis is performed. The hepatic flexure of the colon and small bowel mesentery is mobilized. The pancreas should be uniformly pale yellow, with no tissue edema and minimal tissue trauma. The entire duodenum and pancreas are mobilized by an extended Kocher maneuver, with the division of the ligament of Treitz. The supraceliac aorta is encircled with umbilical tape for aortic cross-clamp after division of the diaphragmatic crura. The IMA is divided between ligatures, and the distal aorta is encircled with umbilical tape. The gastrocolic ligament is divided, and the spleen is mobilized by incising the lateral peritoneal reflection and the splenic flexure. The gastroepiploic and short gastric vessels are dissected and divided between suture ligatures. The porta hepatis is dissected, and the proper hepatic artery and the common bile duct are ligated and divided separately, leaving the portal vein intact. Prior to the ligation of the common bile duct, a Prolene suture is placed on the antimesenteric border of the duodenum to mark the position of the ampulla of Vater by passing a probe down the common bile duct. The common hepatic artery is isolated to its origin. The left gastric artery is identified, ligated, and transected. The splenic artery is identified and encircled at the celiac trunk. Dissection of the hepatic and splenic arteries is minimized to avoid vasospasm. Mobilization of the pancreas laterally to medially in the region of the portal vein is aided by using the spleen as a handle to minimize trauma to the delicate pancreas and to avoid posttransplant pancreatitis. All divided structures in the retroperitoneal area are ligated. The IMV is ligated at the distal margin of the pancreas.

Heparin is given and the systemic circulation is arrested by clamping the supraceliac aorta. The IVC and portal vein are incised, and cold UW solution is introduced through the aortic cannula to perfuse the pancreas and kidneys. The celiac trunk and SMA are excised with a patch from the aorta. The inferior pancreaticoduodenal arteries, which originate from the SMA, must be preserved. The SMV is transected as it enters the pancreas and ligated.

The duodenal lumen, previously irrigated with 500 ml of 20% betadine and/ or amphotericin B (50 mg/L) solution through a nasogastric tube, is transected using a gastrointestinal (GIA) stapler 4 to 6 cm proximal and distal to the previously marked ampulla of Vater. The mesenteric vessels at the inferior border of the pancreas are divided using a GIA stapler. The duodenum is opened and the lumen is irrigated with amphotericin B solution (50 mg/L). The pancreatic graft, duodenum, and spleen are then removed (Fig. 9.3). A bifurcated iliac vessel is harvested for transplantation. The external iliac artery is anastomosed to the SMA and the internal iliac artery, to the splenic artery.

9.3.2. Pancreas with Liver Procurement

The main technical difference is isolating the vascular supply to both organs. The gastroduodenal artery is ligated when the common hepatic and hepatic arteries are needed for the liver, without compromising the blood supply to the head of the pancreas. In most cases, it is preferable to keep the entire hepatic artery with the liver graft, the most common hepatic arterial anomalies being a replaced right hepatic (accessory) artery originating from the SMA in the hepatoduodenal ligament inferior and lateral to the common bile duct. If present, this is divided at the origin of the SMA at the take-off of the right hepatic artery. A replaced left hepatic artery originating from the left gastric artery in the gastrohepatic ligament,

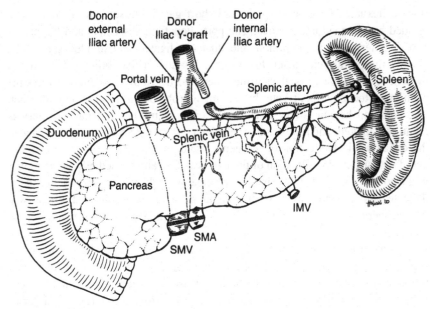

Figure 9.3. Anterior view: The pancreas is prepared by splenectomy and ligation of the splenic artery and superior mesenteric artery (SMA) and vein (SMV), and the duodenal stump is transected with GIA staples and reinforced with Lembert silk sutures.

if present, is isolated and preserved. Liver preparation is described in an earlier section of this chapter. The IMV is isolated and cannulated for portal perfusion. After the supraceliac aorta is cross-clamped, 2 l of cold UW solution is introduced through each of the IMV and distal aortic cannulas.

Upon completion of organ perfusion, the splenic artery is ligated and divided several millimeters distal to its take-off from the celiac trunk; the aorta is divided above and below the origin of the celiac trunk, and the portal vein is divided 2 cm above the superior border of the pancreas. The SMA is divided distal to the origin of interior pancreaticoduodenal artery with an aortic Carrel patch. An iliac arterial graft is obtained from the donor, with the external iliac artery anastomosed to the SMA, and the internal iliac artery is anastomosed to the splenic artery of the pancreatic graft *ex vivo*.

9.4. LIVING DONOR PANCREATECTOMY

The living related pancreas transplantation was pioneered at the University of Minnesota. The procedure has not been without complications. Some of the donors have become diabetic themselves following hemipancreatectomy. Briefly, a bilateral subcostal incision is performed and the gastrocolic omentum is divided, preserving the epiploic vascular arcade and short gastric vessels. The splenic artery and vein are isolated and suture ligated near the splenic hilum. Care is taken to preserve the spleen. The dissection is carried out to the pancreatic neck, at the confluence of the splenic and SMV (i.e., the origin of the portal vein). The splenic vein is isolated and encircled at its termination in the portal vein. The splenic artery, at the origin of the celiac trunk, is identified behind the pancreatic neck and encircled. Heparin (40 U/kg) is given and the splenic vessels at the origin are transected. The pancreas is divided over the portal vein and then removed and flushed with heparinized cold UW solution on the backtable. The splenic vessels are oversewn on the donor, as are the pancreatic duct and the cut surface of the proximal pancreas. A drain is placed in the pancreatic bed, and the abdomen is closed in the usual fashion.

Part III

Recipient Operative Techniques and Strategies

Chapter 10

The Liver Transplant Procedure

Cosme Manzarbeitia and Sukru Emre

10.1. INTRODUCTION

Liver transplantation is often claimed to be the most complex and difficult of all general surgical operations. It is of paramount importance that meticulous and delicate surgical technique be utilized throughout the donor and recipient operative procedures. As in any transplant operation, close attention must constantly be given to methods that minimize trauma and ischemia to the organ during implantation. The surgical techniques for implantation vary depending on whether a whole or partial organ is going to be used, and whether the old liver is totally or partially removed.

Using University of Wisconsin (UW) preservation solution, cold storage can now be maintained for up to 20 hours, with the expectation of prompt function in the recipient, although most centers try to limit the cold ischemic period to 14–15 hours. This allows for both a well-planned surgical procedure and, frequently, the opportunity to perform frozen-section liver biopsy in cases where there is a question about the quality of the donor organ. Only when the liver has received final approval from the recipient surgeon is the patient brought to the operating room and anesthesia initiated. Prior to implantation, the donor liver is removed from the ice cooler and prepared for implantation on a backtable. The extraneous tissues that accompany organs removed en-bloc are trimmed. Arterial reconstruction, if necessary, is performed at this time. The essential principle of arterial reconstruction is to provide a single common inflow vessel, so that only one anastomosis need be performed in the recipient. All vessels are then tested for patency and integrity by flushing with sterile preservation solution. The iliac arteries and veins routinely procured at the termination of the donor operation are prepared for use, if necessary, as venous or arterial grafts in the recipient.

10.2. WHOLE ORGAN IMPLANTATION

10.2.1. Orthotopic Liver Transplantation (OLT)

The basic objective of an OLT operation is to remove the diseased native organ and then replace it in exactly the same location with a normal new one. This recipient hepatectomy may be fraught with the hazard of massive bleeding, increasing subsequent morbidity and mortality. Therefore, it is imperative that careful attention to the meticulous, gentle handling of tissues and a strict systematic approach to hemostasis be followed throughout the recipient operation. Cannulation for bypass is performed percutaneously by the anesthesia team in most cases, using the left saphenous vein and the left internal jugular vein as the sites of choice.

10.2.1.1. Hepatectomy and Bypass

A bilateral subcostal incision with a midline extension to the xiphoid process is routinely used. After dividing the round and falciform ligaments, a large, self-retaining upper abdominal retractor is placed, which aids greatly in the exposure of the entire liver and, more importantly, the suprahepatic vena cava. The ligamentous attachments of the liver are then dissected, including the left and right triangular ligaments, as well as the gastrohepatic ligament. The hilar dissection then proceeds (Fig. 10.1), with systematic ligation of the hepatic artery, cystic duct, and common hepatic duct. The portal vein is then cleaned of surrounding neurolymphatic tissue from the level of the head of the pancreas up to its bifurcation. The hepatic artery is now formally dissected, exposing the common hepatic artery to allow for subsequent anastomosis.

Venovenous bypass may now be initiated (Fig. 10.2). The decision when to go on bypass depends on the degree of portal hypertension, the extent of previous surgery with vascularized adhesions, and the degree of bleeding from the raw surface of the liver. In some cases, especially in patients with cholestatic liver disease and no previous surgery, the entire mobilization and dissection of the liver can be done prior to the institution of the venovenous bypass. However, in cases with severe portal hypertension and previous surgery in which bleeding was a problem, venovenous bypass should be initiated at the earliest opportunity.

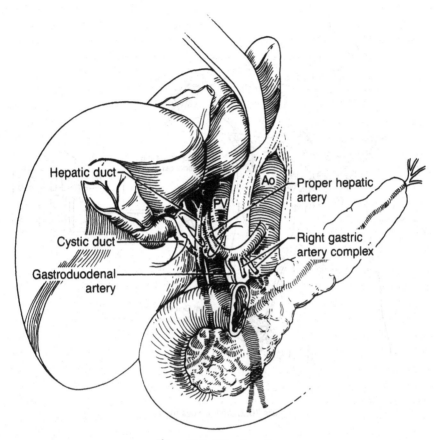

Figure 10.1. Hilar dissection

10.2.1.2. Anhepatic Phase and Donor Liver Implantation

The remaining attachments to the liver can be divided rapidly once the liver has been completely devascularized. The liver is then sharply excised (Fig. 10.3), leaving an upper caval cuff at the diaphragm that includes the open orifices of the hepatic veins, a lower caval cuff above the renal veins, and the bare area that was behind the right lobe of the liver. The bare area is oversewn for hemostasis (Fig. 10.4), and the vena caval cuff is fashioned for anastomosis.

The implantation of the liver follows a strict routine. The suprahepatic vena cava is anastomosed first. With this completed, the vena cava is anastomosed below the liver; a venting catheter is left within the cava through the lower caval

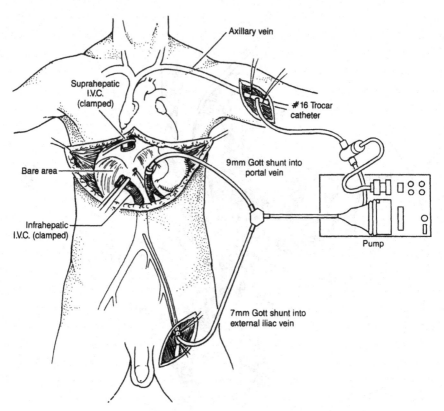

Figure 10.2. Venovenous bypass.

anastomosis, which is left untied until after reperfusion. The recipient portal vein is now decannulated. The donor and recipient portal veins are then anastomosed in a manner that redundancy and kinking are avoided. The liver is then flushed free of preservation solution prior to reopening the circulation by infusion of a crystalloid solution via the portal vein during the infrahepatic vena caval anastomosis or with portal blood subsequent to the portal anastomosis. After reperfusion, the caval clamps are opened, restoring normal flow. A rapid inspection for hemostasis is made, and attention is turned to the hepatic artery. We have found that the routine use of the common hepatic artery at the level of the gastroduodenal is the most common source of adequate inflow, and avoids a duodenal steal phenomenon. The anastomosis is performed in an end-to-end fashion, sewing the common hepatic artery to the celiac artery of the donor. To confirm adequacy of the arterial reconstruction, flow is measured with an electromagnetic flow meter at the completion of the vascular anastomoses. If flow is found to be inadequate, the artery is scrutinized to determine the reason and any problems are corrected. If there is any

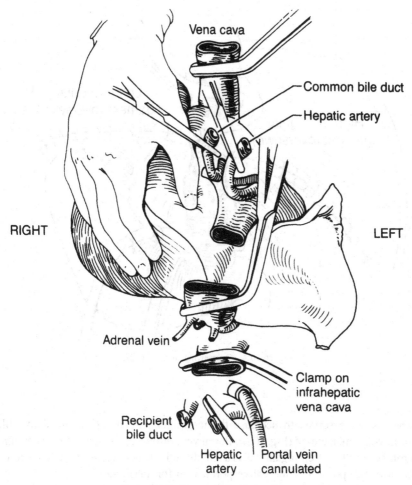

Figure 10.3. Removal of recipient liver.

doubt as to the adequacy of the inflow, an aortohepatic graft should be fashioned by utilizing donor iliac artery. Grafts can be also used to lengthen the vessels for anastomosis as interposition arterial or venous grafts (Fig. 10.5). The graft is then sewn end-to-end to the celiac axis of the donor liver.

10.2.1.3. The Problem of Portal Vein Thrombosis

Techniques for the replacement of the portal vein or for thrombectomy of a recent thrombosis have been described. The use of donor iliac vein grafts from the superior mesenteric vein, tunneled toward the hepatic hilum over the neck of the

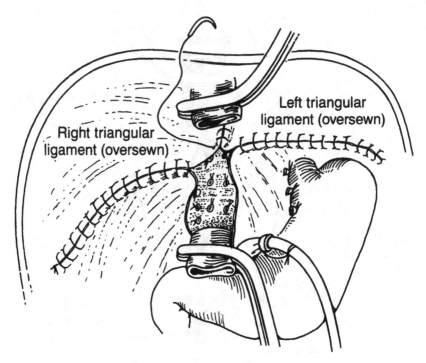

Figure 10.4. Oversewing of bare areas.

pancreas, have served to decrease the morbidity and mortality attendant with portal vein replacement (Fig. 10.6). Portal vein thrombectomy, in cases where the thrombosis is less well organized, is a simple and effective technique that reserves the proximal portion of the native portal vein for anastomosis.

10.2.1.4.   Hemostasis Period, Biliary Reconstruction, and Closure

Prior to the reestablishment of biliary continuity, hemostasis must be complete. While, in some cases, this task may consist of the simple inspection of the anastomoses and suture of a few small bleeding points, in other cases, it may require tremendous effort to control bleeding completely. Once achieved, the biliary reconstruction can begin. Biliary reconstruction, once considered the Achilles' heel of liver transplantation, is now a routine and simple procedure. If the recipient bile duct is of normal caliber and free of intrinsic disease, a simple donor-to-recipient, duct-to-duct reconstruction can be performed over an indwelling T-tube stent (Fig. 10.7B) that is exteriorized through a separate stab wound

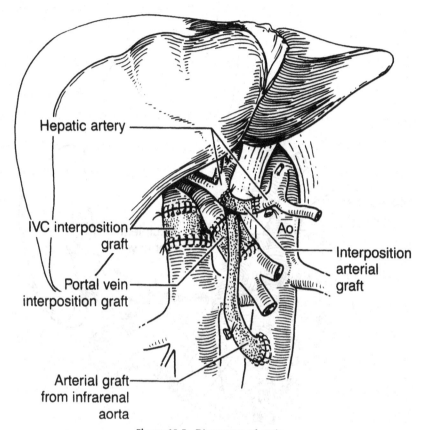

Hepatic artery

IVC interposition graft

Portal vein interposition graft

Ao

Interposition arterial graft

Arterial graft from infrarenal aorta

Figure 10.5. Diverse use of grafts.

incision. The T tube acts not only as a stent to prevent possible stricture but also prevents kinking. If the two ends of the bile duct can be tailored to meet perfectly without redundancy and are of similar caliber, this end-to-end reconstruction can be performed without a T tube. This eliminates the potential complication of bile leakage from the point where the T tube exits the duct that may occur when the T tube is removed 3 months posttransplant. If the patient's native bile duct is diseased, or if the duct is too small, the bile duct of the donor is anastomosed to a defunctionalized Roux-en-Y loop of jejunum over an internal stent (Fig. 10.7A). In these cases, percutaneous methods must be used to visualize the bile duct.

Cholangiography is performed to confirm a technically sound biliary reconstruction and may be performed through the T tube or via the cystic duct. The anastomosis should appear widely patent and without leaks. With this completed, closing the abdomen after leaving three closed suction drains above and below the liver concludes the operation.

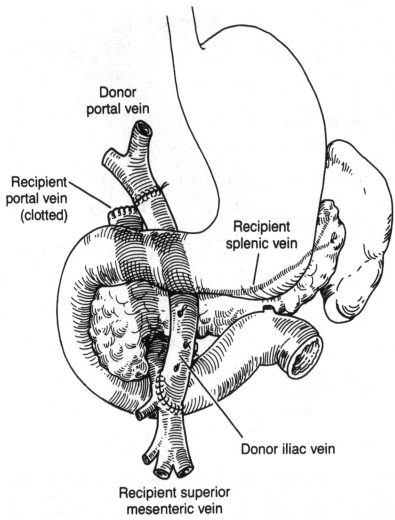

Figure 10.6. Jump graft, portal vein.

10.2.2. Piggyback Techniques

In certain cases, removal of the cava is not necessary. In these cases, leaving the recipient's cava in place and dissecting the caudate lobe off the cava by dividing the short hepatic veins individually preserves the caval continuity. This leaves the liver attached by the three main hepatic veins. These are controlled with a clamp, and a common cuff fashioned from the orifices of the three veins, which

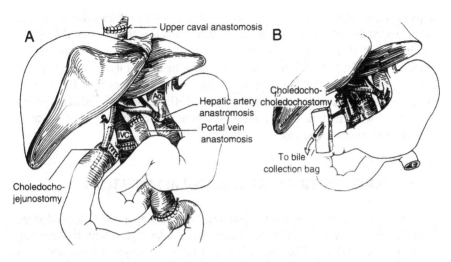

Figure 10.7. The final result.

in turn is anastomosed to the donor liver's suprahepatic cava. Bypass, either total or partial (only portal flow diverted), may be instituted or omitted altogether. If bypass is omitted, this is accomplished either by creating a temporary portocaval shunt or by simply clamping the portal vein, if the hemodynamic status of the patient allows it. There is no need to perform a lower caval anastomosis, and the donor infrahepatic cava is tied or stapled shut. The rest of the case proceeds as described earlier.

10.3. Heterotopic/Auxiliary Transplantation

Heterotopic liver transplantation techniques (HLT) leave the native liver in place. They have not found wide acceptance in cases of chronic end-stage liver disease due to various clinical issues, including the excellent results with OLT, the late presentation of hepatocellular carcinoma in the cirrhotic native liver, physical space considerations, and functional blood flow competition issues.

HLT has been occasionally used in cases of fulminant liver failure (FHF), in which attempts at removal of the native liver led to prohibitive increases in intracranial pressure. In these cases, the liver is often implanted in a location different from the native liver location. HLT in FHF cases has the appeal of leaving the native liver in place, which may allow for late regeneration of the liver and eventual withdrawal of immunosuppression. Technical points that should be considered include reduction in graft size, graft perfusion with portal venous and hepatic arterial flow, and hepatic venous drainage of the draft into the suprarenal vena cava of the recipient. A serious concern is whether the low portal pressure would preferentially shunt portal blood flow to the native liver and threaten the viability of the HLT graft. Thus, a constriction or ligation of the portal vein in the native liver may be mandatory for graft viability in the absence of portal hypertension. Techniques that have been described for FHF include reduced-size heterotopic graft, with right subhepatic location (Moritz), and auxiliary partial orthotopic liver transplantation (APOLT) (Pichlmayr).

10.4. PARTIAL/SEGMENTAL ORGAN IMPLANTATION

While liver transplantation has become the treatment of choice for end-stage liver disease, the number of organ donors has not kept pace with the growing number of candidates. The increasing gap between supply and demand has resulted in higher mortality among candidates on the waiting list. In attempts to narrow this gap, transplant centers have broadened their donor selection criteria and have begun to employ innovative surgical techniques (see Fig. 10.8), such as reduced-size liver transplantation, split-liver transplantation, and living donor liver transplantation.

10.4.1. Reduced-Size Liver Transplantation

This technique was introduced in the mid-1980s in order to provide size-matched grafts for pediatric patients. In reduced-size liver transplantation, a cadaveric liver procured using standard techniques is resected on the backtable to craft a smaller-sized graft. The liver allograft can be tailored based on the recipient's body size. It is possible to create a right-lobe graft, a left-lobe graft, or a left lateral segment graft. The rest of the liver is discarded.

10.4.2. Split-Liver Transplantation

This technique was an outgrowth of reduced-size liver transplantation and was first employed in 1988 in Europe. This technique is appealing because it provides two allografts from a single donor liver, thus increasing the number of available grafts.

10.4.2.1. Anatomical Considerations

In split-liver transplantation, a whole adult liver is transected into two pieces to provide grafts for two recipients. The splitting procedure can be done through

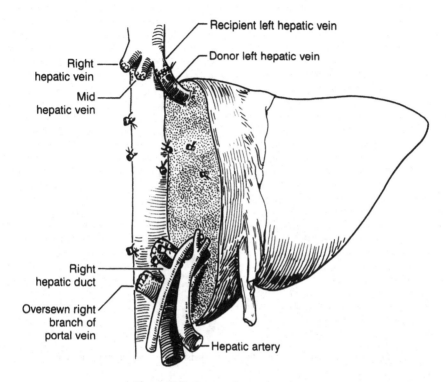

Figure 10.8. Segmental transplantation.

the falciform ligament to provide a small (left lateral segment) graft for a child and a large (extended right lobe) graft for an adult. It is also possible to split a whole liver through the main portal fissure to create right-lobe (segments I and VI–VIII) and left-lobe (segments II, III, and IV) grafts (Fig. 10.9).

10.4.2.2. Surgical Technique

Liver splitting can be done *ex situ* or *in situ*. In an *ex situ* fashion, the liver is split on the backtable after the organ has been procured using standard techniques (see Chapter 8). In the *in situ* procedure, splitting is performed in the donor before aortic clamping, while the heart is still beating. Technically, the procedure is similar to living donor liver transplantation, as described below.

10.4.2.3. Left Lateral Segment Splitting (ex situ)

After a standard backtable procedure is performed, the left hepatic artery is dissected out, from its origin to the umbilical fissure. The left portal vein as well

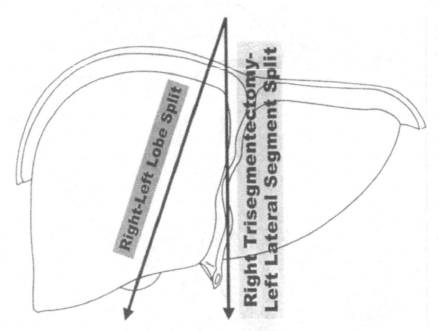

Figure 10.9. Anatomical lines for hepatic division in split-liver transplantation.

is freed up from its bifurcation to the level of umbilical fissure. After this is completed, the left hepatic vein is isolated and divided. The left hepatic vein orifice on the cava is closed vertically using 5/0 prolene running suture. The parenchymal transsection line is to the right side of the falciform ligament; parenchymal transsection is performed using scissor dissection. The vascular and bile duct branches are tied and divided. During the parenchymal transection, the portal vein branches supplying the left medial segment (segment 4) must be transected, sometimes causing necrosis of segment 4. When liver splitting is performed *ex situ*, the viability of segment 4 should be evaluated after the liver is reperfused, and segment 4 should be resected if it becomes dusky following reperfusion.

   In situ splitting has many advantages over *ex situ* splitting. Because no backtable liver division is needed with *in situ* procurement, so-called cool ischemia is avoided. The vascular supply of segment 4 can be evaluated. Because bleeding and bile leakage from the cut edge are controlled during parenchymal dissection, bleeding from the raw surface on reperfusion is minimal. One part of the liver can be shipped to another center directly from the donor hospital, avoiding extended cold-ischemia time and facilitating intercenter sharing.

   In both *in situ* and *ex situ* splitting, vessels can be shared based on both recipients' needs. For example, because the hepatic artery is small in pediatric patients, especially those below 1 year of age, it would be ideal to leave the whole celiac axis with the left lateral segment graft, so that the donor celiac axis can be anastomosed to the infrarenal aorta without an extension graft. On the other hand, in adults, the right hepatic artery of the donor can easily be anastomosed to the recipient's right or proper hepatic artery without using operating microscope, since the diameter of the right hepatic artery is generally > 3 mm. In terms of portal vein sharing, the donor's left portal vein is usually long enough to reach the bifurcation of the recipient's portal vein without an extension graft; thus, the main portal vein usually remains with the right graft.

10.4.2.4. Donor Selection Criteria for Split-Liver Transplantation

Although donor acceptance criteria have been broadened for whole-liver transplantation (in terms of age, cardiac arrest, and pressor support), for split-liver transplantation these criteria are still strict, since graft-associated problems are multiplied when a liver is split for two recipients. Donor age ideally is < 50 years, and donors should be in the hospital < 3 days, with perfect liver function, minimal pressor support, and no steatosis. The final decision of whether a liver is suitable for splitting should be made in the operating room after assessment of the liver by an experienced surgeon.

10.4.2.5. Recipient Selection Criteria

Recipient selection criteria are also important for split-liver transplantation, especially for adult recipients. It is believed that relatively stable patients better tolerate split-related complications. The best results with this technique have been achieved when the grafts were allocated to stable Child's B-C patients. Recently, using *in situ* splitting technique, split grafts have been successfully used in high-risk recipients.

10.4.3. Living Donor Liver Transplantation

In living donor liver transplantation, another innovative technique, part of the liver from a living donor is resected and transplanted into a recipient. The technique was first used for pediatric recipients in order to overcome the shortage of small liver allografts. Because results have been excellent, with established donor safety, living donor liver transplants are now being offered to adult recipients. In pediatric recipients younger than age 5, the left lateral segment of adult liver usually provides a size-matched allograft. For teenage recipients, a left lobe should be used. For adults, right lobe grafts are necessary to ensure enough liver volume. More than 2,000 living donor operations have been performed worldwide. Although the donor operation has been associated with low morbidity and mortality, long-term follow-up is necessary to confirm the safety of this procedure for donors, especially for donors of the right lobe grafts.

Because this procedure subjects a healthy individual (the donor) to major surgery, donor safety is essential and informed consent is crucial. The American Society of Transplant Surgeons (ASTS) has published guidelines for living donor transplantation. The risks and benefits of the living donor operation must be explained to the donor, to the recipient, and to their immediate families. In addition, donors should be thoroughly evaluated by an unbiased physician. The workup should include a history and physical, chest X-ray, electrocardiogram (EKG), blood work (including liver functions and viral serologies), and magnetic resonance imaging (MRI) with calculation of liver volume.

The procedure provides many advantages to the recipient. The transplant operation can be done electively, without having to wait for a cadaveric organ, before the recipient develops serious complications of end-stage liver disease. Furthermore, since the donor is healthy and ischemia time is short, graft quality is better than with cadaveric liver allografts. The recipient and donor operations are performed simultaneously, or in an overlapping fashion, to minimize ischemia time. Technical problems in the recipient, such as hepatic artery thrombosis and biliary leaks were seen initially but have decreased dramatically with increasing experience in technique and recipient selection. For the donors, the advantage is mainly psychological.

The liver rapidly regenerates in both donors and recipients, and normal liver volume is almost completely restored. Although this process takes 6–8 weeks, most of the regeneration occurs within the first 2 weeks following the procedure.

10.4.4. Recipient Operation for Split-Liver and Living Donor Grafts

The operation to implant a right lobe split graft is similar to whole-liver OLT (see previous discussion). In the case of left or left-lateral segment split grafts, and all living donor liver grafts, the allograft does not have the vena cava, and therefore the upper caval anastomosis is done using the piggyback technique (Fig. 10.10). The portal vein anastomosis is done between the allograft portal vein and the recipient portal vein using 6-0 Prolene continuous suture. The hepatic artery anastomosis is performed between the allograft hepatic artery (either right or left) and the recipient right or left hepatic artery using 8-0 Prolene interrupted sutures. In pediatric recipients, an operating microscope is necessary for arterial anastomoses. When the entire length of the recipient portal vein and hepatic artery is

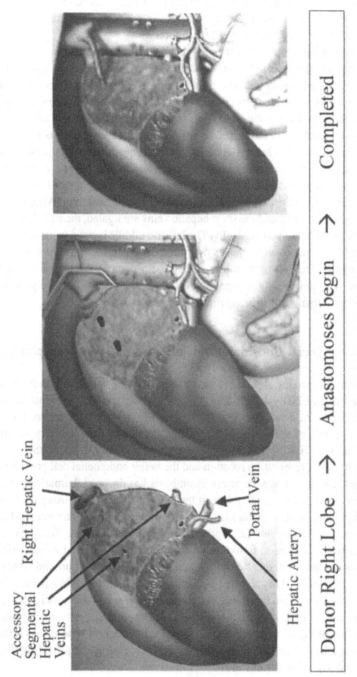

Accessory Segmental Hepatic Veins

Right Hepatic Vein

Portal Vein

Hepatic Artery

Donor Right Lobe → Anastomoses begin → Completed

Figure 10.10. Implantation of right lobe using piggyback technique.

dissected into the hilum, extension grafts are rarely needed. In the majority of cases, bile duct anastomosis is done by Roux-en-Y hepaticojejunostomy using interrupted 6-0 polydiaxanone (PDS) sutures.

The implantation used is the piggyback technique, as follows: For left hemi-grafts, the liver is dissected off the cava, the short hepatic veins are ligated, and the hepatic veins are identified. The right hepatic vein is clamped and divided, and oversewn with 5-0 Prolene sutures. The left and middle hepatic veins are clamped, and the diseased liver is removed. The bridge between the left and middle hepatic veins is transected to make a single orifice. Since the vena cava is not clamped, venous return to the heart is not hampered. The donor suprahepatic cava is anastomosed to the common orifice of the left and middle hepatic veins using 4-0 Prolene running sutures. For right lobe adult-to-adult living donor liver transplan-tation, performing the upper caval anastomoses is quite different. After the liver is dissected off the cava and the short hepatic veins are ligated, the right hepatic vein is encircled and clamped vertically. The left and middle hepatic veins are clamped, and the liver is removed by transecting these three hepatic veins flush on the liver parenchyma. The left and middle hepatic vein orifices are oversewn with 5-0 Prolene. The donor's right hepatic vein is anastomosed to the recipient's right hepatic vein using 5-0 Prolene running suture.

10.4.5.   Special Considerations in Pediatric Liver Transplantation

In addition to the aforementioned issues, liver transplantation in the pediatric population, especially in children weighing 10 kg or less, presents numerous challenges to the transplant team. Vascular thrombosis is common due to the diminutive size of the vessels. Historically, the rate of hepatic artery thrombosis was as high as 20% or 30% in babies weighing less than 10 kg. With the routine use of the UW preservation solution and the better endothelial cell preservation it provides, the rate of hepatic artery thrombosis has dropped dramatically but still remains a significant problem. One of the hidden advantages in using the reduced-size segmental grafts in babies is that their arteries are long and large, and can be anastomosed directly to the supraceliac or infrarenal aorta. This type of re-vascularization has been found to have a lower rate of arterial thrombosis, pre-sumably because of the better inflow and larger anastomosis possible due to the size of the vessels. Many children with biliary atresia are found to have very small, atretic portal veins and large venous collaterals. The use of this small native portal vein for inflow is problematic, and liberal use of venous grafts arising from the confluence of the splenic and superior mesenteric veins is wise in this group. In this way, a large, spatulated anastomosis can be constructed, providing the liver graft with vigorous portal inflow.

The final major hurdle in pediatric liver transplantation is also most prominently found in babies with biliary atresia. Because almost all of these children have had previous portoenterostomy (Kasai) procedures that may have required multiple revisions, the recipient hepatectomy can be extraordinarily difficult; occasionally, enterotomies are inadvertently made because of the extensive nature of the adhesions and their vascularity. Most often, damaged areas are recognized and repaired at the time of surgery, but occasionally small bowel segments become devascularized, leading to the syndrome of multiple bowel fistulae in the postoperative period, a most difficult clinical problem. Therefore, the preference of all pediatric liver transplant surgeons is that Kasai-type procedures be performed only once, so as to avoid these very difficult problems when it is clear that the ultimate step of liver transplantation will be necessary.

Chapter **11**

The Kidney Transplant Procedure
Shuin-Lin Yang

11.1. BACKTABLE GRAFT PREPARATION

In preparation for implantation, the kidney is unpackaged and transferred from the preservation fluid container to a backtable basin full of icy Ringer's lactate solution. The preservation fluid is cultured, as a guide for potential latent infection therapy at a later date. The perirenal fat and the adrenal gland are dissected off the kidney. The surgeon then checks and ligates all open ends from small branches of vessels and lymphatics, to avoid postreperfusion bleeding and posttransplant lymphocele formation.

The dissection of the vessels then proceeds. In left kidney grafts, the renal vein usually is longer, and sometimes comes with or without a vena cava cuff. The gonadal, adrenal, and occasional lumbar vein branches are divided and ligated. After trimming the open end to proper size, no further reconstruction is necessary. In right grafts, most of the time, the kidney comes with a piece or a segment of vena cava; if the renal vein proper is too short, several techniques for the reconstruction of vena cava with sutures or staplers can extend the length of the right renal vein. In grafts with multiple veins, if there is a dominant vein, the smaller vein can be ligated off without compromising the circulation; if both veins are equal caliber, they can sometimes be joined together into a single channel for anastomosis. The right renal vein of the living donor kidney can be short, but usually no reconstruction is done, since there is no vena cava cuff available.

As for the arteries, in cadaveric donors with single arteries, a Carrel patch can be tailored from the aortic cuff to prevent stenosis of arterial anastomosis. For those grafts with multiple arteries, if the arteries are very close together, all the orifices can be included in a single Carrel patch. If the arteries are far apart from each other, they can be reconstructed by joining two patches together to form a single patch. The renal arteries of living donor kidneys are usually short and always lack an aortic patch. When there are multiple arteries, these can either be prepared for implantation separately, or, to shorten warm ischemia time during anastomosis, be reconstructed side-by-side into a common lumen; the end of one artery to the side of another; or joined individually to a common venous patch, harvested from the gonadal vein of the donor kidney.

As for the ureter, caution must be exercised to avoid too much dissection of surrounding tissue, which can compromise the vascular supply of the ureter and might cause ischemic complications after implantation.

Finally, flushing cold Ringer's solution through the vessels before implantation will flush out the high concentration of potassium and also help to identify any vascular structural defects or leaks.

11.2. RECIPIENT SURGERY

11.2.1. Position and Preparation

The patient is placed in the supine position with both arms extended. A Foley catheter is then inserted using full sterile technique, and the urinary bladder is filled with antibiotic solution (e.g., 80 mg Gentamycin in 250 cc normal saline). The Foley catheter is then connected to the urinary bag, and a heavy clamp is applied to the tube to retain the solution in the bladder.

11.2.2. Incision at Lower Quadrant of Abdomen

A curvilinear (hockey stick-shaped) incision is made on either side of lower abdomen, depending on the history of previous surgery or the plan for pancreas transplant, if any. The incision is made from the midline about 1–2 fingerbreadths superior to the pubic tubercle, and extended laterally and superiorly. Some surgeons prefer to incise at the lateral border of the rectus sheath, while others prefer to incise to the oblique and transversalis muscle layers more laterally.

11.2.3. Retroperitoneal Space Dissection

The retroperitoneal space is then entered after incising the transversalis fascia. The peritoneal sac and its contents are then retracted medially to expose the iliac vessels and make room for the implanted kidney. In female patients, the round ligament usually can be divided after ligation to gain more exposure. In male patients, the spermatic cord has to be preserved; injury to this structure can lead to testicular atrophy or hydrocele formation.

11.2.4. Isolation of Iliac Vessels

The inferior epigastric vessels may be divided to gain better exposure. The lymphatics surrounding the iliac vessels need to be ligated before division to prevent posttransplant lymphocele formation; use of electrocauterization in this area is usually less effective in preventing this. The dissection of iliac vessels should be limited distally to the area cephalad to the inguinal lymph nodes. The proximal dissection should be limited to the bifurcation of external and internal iliac arteries. Minimizing the area of dissection reduces the incidence of post-transplant lymphocele formation. The external iliac artery seldom has branches in this area; it can be encircled with soft, rubber vessel loops and mobilized freely. The iliac vein dissection sometimes includes the complete division of all hypo-gastric veins to ensure the mobility and exposure of the external iliac vein. This is particularly true in the left iliac vein, which is usually located much more posterior in comparison to the right iliac vein.

11.2.5. Vascular Anastomosis

The venous anastomosis is usually performed first. After total control of external iliac vein is achieved proximally and distally, a longitudinal venotomy is made in the side of the donor's renal vein opening. The anastomosis is then fashioned with 5-0 Prolene running sutures. The traditional arterial anastomosis with the internal iliac artery has the advantage of gaining some length from the internal iliac artery to overcome the shortness of the donor renal artery, partic-ularly in a living kidney donor. This, however, requires more extensive dissection and ligation of the internal iliac artery, with various potential complications. Most surgeons prefer anastomosis to the external iliac artery in end-to-side fashion. When there are multiple arteries, a Carrel patch can be fashioned to include all the arteries in one patch, if the arteries are close enough in a cadaveric donor kidney. If the arteries are far apart or in a living donor kidney, then arterial reconstructions at the backtable will be needed. If both arteries are of equal size, they can be joined to the external iliac artery separately. In order to reduce the warm ischemic time during the arterial anastomosis, various techniques of arterial reconstruction can be performed at the backtable, as described earlier. Sometimes a small upper pole artery can be sacrificed, if it is too small for reconstruction; on the other hand, the lower pole artery is very important to the arterial blood supply of the ureter, so reconstruction should always be attempted. Usually, prosthetic materials (e.g., Gore-Tex) are not recommended for reconstruction.

Mannitol and furosemide are given just prior to releasing the vascular clamps for reperfusion. Upon reperfusion, hemostasis should be obtained by careful inspection of both anastomoses and ligation of all bleeders at small branches of the vessels. Warm irrigation fluid should be applied to help warm up the kidney. The kidney usually becomes firm and pink a few minutes are revascularization. The urine may begin to flow out of the ureter soon thereafter, particularly if the ischemia time was minimal. If the kidney remains flaccid after reperfusion, careful inspections of external iliac and renal arteries should rule out any arterial inflow problems. The systemic pressure and the central venous pressure must be maintained at an adequate level to ensure proper renal perfusion pressure. If vasospasm is suspected, papaverine or verapamil may be injected into the transplanted renal artery. If after all these measures the kidney is still flaccid and not producing urine, then the transplant kidney may be suffering from delayed graft function. Very rarely, hyperacute rejection should be considered as a possibility. A needle biopsy and/or wedge biopsy is taken at this point as the baseline histology control to be used for comparison in future biopsies.

11.2.6.   Ureteric Reconstruction and Closure

In female patients, the round ligament is usually transected to gain exposure, and the ureter can be brought down to the urinary bladder directly. In the male patient, the ureter will be passed underneath the spermatic cord to the urinary bladder. The rectus muscle might need to be partially transected and the urinary bladder distended with irrigation solution to help the dissection of the fat tissue anterior to the urinary bladder, and to expose the dome of the bladder for urinary reconstruction. Once the proper location has been identified, the surgeon proceeds with the ureteroneocystostomy using one of two techniques. In the modified *Lich–Gregoir procedure* (extravesical), the detrusor muscle is incised for about 3 cm with electrocauterization to expose the underneath mucosal layer. A small cystostomy is made and confirmed by noticing the flow of the previously instilled antibiotic solution. The heavy clamp on the Foley tube is then removed. Stay stitches are placed on each side to help exposure of the cystostomy. The ureter is shortened to adequate length, and the end is spatulated to match the bladder opening. A mucosa-to-mucosa anastomosis is performed with 5-0 polydiaxanone (PDS), monocryl or vicryl. The detrusor muscle layer is then closed over the ureter to form a submucosal tunnel as an antireflux measure. As an alternative technique (single-stitch technique), two parallel incisions are made on the bladder wall down to the submucosal layer; the ureter is passed from the first to the second incision through a submucosal tunnel, and the ureteral implantation is performed at the level of the second incision. A single anchor stitch is applied to secure the ureter.

The *Ledbetter–Politano procedure* (transvesical) is considered by some surgeons to more effectively prevent vesicoureteral reflux. In this technique, the surgeon creates an anterior cystotomy and, working within the bladder, pulls the ureter through a submucosal tunnel into the bladder, performing the anastomosis near the base of the bladder. The cystostomy is then closed in layers. In either procedure, some centers routinely insert a double "J" stent, to be removed a few weeks later, to ensure the patency of the anastomosis.

When the donor ureter is too short to reach the urinary bladder, an *uretero-ureterostomy* or *ureteropyelostomy* may be needed. In these techniques, the recipient's native ureter is utilized for reconstruction. After careful dissection of the ureter to avoid devascularization, the proximal end of the ureter is ligated and its distal end is then spatulated for anastomosis to either the donor ureter or to the pelvis of the donor kidney, respectively. If the patient is still making urine, an ipsilateral nephrectomy may be required to prevent hydronephrosis and possible infection. In both techniques, a double "J" ureteral stent is often required to prevent urinary fistula or stricture formation.

In cases with double ureters, both ureters can either be reconstructed into a common opening or be anastomosed separately to the bladder. In rare instances, a urinary diversion procedure such as an *ileal* or *colonic conduit* may be necessary. Any urinary diversion procedure should be planned and performed long before the transplant. The bowel segment of the conduit should be positioned for easy access. The location of the stoma should be carefully placed so as not to interfere with the transplant incision.

Prior to *closure*, the kidney is placed at the parapsoas fossa to avoid kinking of the vessels or ureter. The incision is then closed in layers with PDS or Prolene sutures. The skin is then closed with staples or sutures. Unless special conditions arise, no drains are used.

Chapter 12

The Pancreas Transplant Procedure

Jorge A. Ortiz

The technique of pancreas transplantation has evolved greatly over the last decade. Exocrine drainage was initially performed via the enteric route or the duct was sclerosed. However, by 1995, 90% of centers were draining by way of the bladder. In the year 2000, the pendulum has swung back. Approximately 50% of pancreata are drained enterically. Similarly, many more centers are providing venous drainage by way of the portal vein instead of the iliac vein, in order to avoid systemic hyperinsulinemia. Additionally, some groups place the organ in the retroperitoneal position as opposed to intra-abdominally. The following is a brief review of the various techniques of pancreas transplantation.

12.1. BACKTABLE PREPARATION

The backtable preparation of the pancreas involves trimming and oversewing of redundant duodenum. The ampulla of Vater must be in plain sight so as not to compromise it. Safe anastomosis necessitates 6–8 cm of duodenum. Fibrofatty tissue surrounding the pancreas is ligated, as are the inferior mesenteric vein, the gastroduodenal artery, and the middle colic vessels. Some groups perform splenectomy on the backtable, while others wait until reperfusion and use the spleen as a handle during the operation. The splenic and superior mesenteric arteries are reconstructed using the donor iliac artery. The internal iliac is anastomosed to the splenic mesenteric artery and the external iliac artery is anastomosed to the superior mesenteric artery (SMA) on the backtable with 5-0 or 6-0 running nonabsorb-

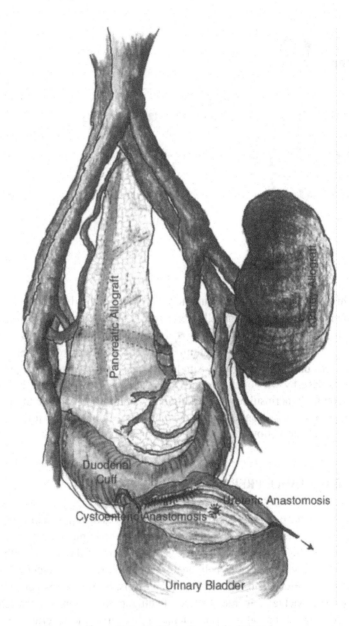

Figure 12.1. Bladder and systemic drainage.

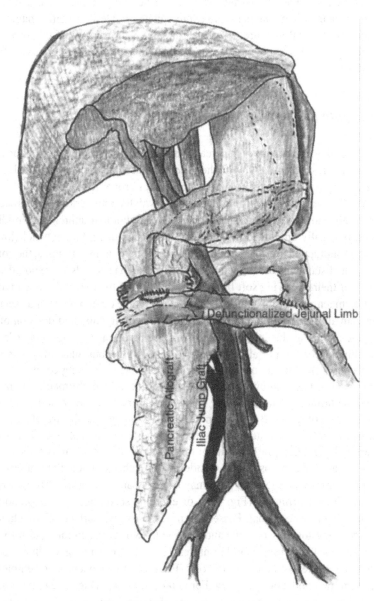

Figure 12.2. Enteric and portal drainage.

able suture. This provides one orifice for subsequent arterial anastomosis on the operating table later on. If there are no suitable iliac grafts, the donor's brachiocephalic trunk can be used. Additionally, the splenic artery may be anastomosed, with or without an interposition graft, end-to-side to the SMA. Placing the portal vein on traction with stay sutures facilitates venous reconstruction. The coronary vein, as well as small tributaries draining the head of the pancreas, should be ligated, as their subsequent tearing may precipitate troublesome hemorrhage. Two centimeters of portal vein are necessary for safe reconstruction. If this is not the case, elongation of the vein can be performed with a jump graft of iliac vein from the cadaver.

12.2. IMPLANTATION PROCEDURE

In simultaneous kidney–pancreas transplantation, the procedure is usually performed intra-abdominally, with the pancreas placed on the right and the kidney on the left. It is also possible to perform bilateral retroperitoneal dissections. It is believed that there may be more complications with the retroperitoneal approaches but they are more easily managed. In the intra-abdominal approach, a midline incision is usually employed, although some centers use a Pfannenstiel (lower, transverse suprapubic muscle-splitting) incision. For systemic drainage, the colon, cecum, and distal ileum are reflected superiorly. The iliac vessels are exposed after removal of their overlying soft tissue. Mobilization of the iliac vein may involve only a 2-cm length of vein anteriorly, or it may involve circumferential dissection of the vein all the way to the inferior vena cava, with ligation and division of all branches, including the internal iliac. Some believe that the subsequent laxity avoids kinking of the portal iliac anastomosis. The venous anastomosis is performed end-to-side, from donor portal vein to the iliac vein, using continuous 5-0 or 6-0 nonabsorbable suture. The arterial anastomosis is performed in a similar end-to-side fashion from the Y graft to the iliac artery. In portal venous drainage, the portal vein of the graft is anastomosed end-to-side to a major tributary of the superior mesenteric vein after lifting the transverse colon cephalad. The donor iliac artery bifurcation graft is brought through a window made in the distal ileal mesentery and anastomosed end-to-side to the right common iliac artery. An innominate artery interposition graft may be necessary to simplify this approach.

For *bladder drainage* (Fig. 12.1) of exocrine secretions, the projection of the pancreas must be caudal. Dissection proceeds on the surface of the bladder. The duodenocystostomy can be hand sewn with two layers, an inner, absorbable suture and an outer nonabsorble suture. This can be running or interrupted. Alternatively, an end-to-end anastomosis (EEA) stapling device can be employed to perform the duodenocystostomy. For *enteric drainage* (Fig. 12.2), the projection of the pancreas can be caudal or cephalad. The transplanted duodenum is anastomosed to a segment of distal ileum or a diverted Roux-en-Y limb of recipient jejunum.

Chapter 13

Anesthesia in Abdominal Organ Transplantation

Jonathan V. Roth and Jan Kramer

13.1. ANESTHETIC MANAGEMENT OF THE ORGAN DONOR

The anesthesiologist is a key member of the recovery team. The goal of management during multiorgan procurements is to maintain physiologic stability (i.e., oxygenation and perfusion), so that the organs will be in the best possible condition when they are harvested. Donors are brain dead and thus do not require an anesthetic, though they may still elicit visceral, somatic, and autonomic reflexes. Additionally, the anesthesiologist may be asked to administer certain medications, such as mannitol, furosemide, and heparin, as part of the organ procurement protocol.

Table 13.1 displays the physiologic derangements most often seen. In general, the goal is to provide supportive care for any of these conditions in order to avoid any insult to the organ(s) to be harvested. The following are points to consider during any given donor's intraoperative management:

- Bradycardia may sometimes be resistant to atropine but respond to direct-acting chronotropic agents (e.g., dopamine or isoproterenol).
- Maintain urine output of at least 1 cc/kg/min. Fluids may be given freely, in joint discussion and accord with the surgical procurement teams. Hypernatremia and polyuria due to diabetes insipidus are managed with volume replacement and vasopressin (0.5–15.0 units/hr).
- Administer pancuronium 0.15–0.20 mg/kg intravenously (IV) to avoid reflex neuromuscular activity.

TABLE 13.1. Physiological Derangements in the Brain Dead Organ Donor

Hypotension	Hypothermia
Hypovolemia (diabetes insipidus, hemorrhage)	Hypothalamic infarction
Neurogenic shock	Exposure
Hypoxemia	Dysrhythmia (especially bradycardia)
Neurogenic pulmonary edema	Intracranial injury or herniation
Pulmonary contusion	Hypothermia
Pneumonia	Hypoxia
Gastric aspiration	Electrolyte abnormality
Fluid overload	Myocardial contusion, ischemia

SOURCES: Firestone L, Firestone S. Anesthesia for organ transplantation. In: *Clinical Anesthesia* (2nd ed.). J. B. Lippincott, Philadelphia, 1992, pp. 1479–1511. Roth JV. Transesophageal pacing and recording: An update. *Progress in Anesthesiology* 1996;X(22):431–448.

- Set ventilator settings to $F_IO_2 = 1$, positive-end expiratory pressure (PEEP) = 2–5 cm H_2O, tidal volume = 10–12 cc/kg, and rate adjusted to maintain $PaCO_2$ = 30–45 torr.
- Maintain the central venous pressure (CVP) between 8–12 cm H_2O for hemodynamic stabilization.
- If after adequate hydration, the CVP is appropriate but the systemic blood pressure (BP) is low (systolic less than 100 mmHg), begin inotrope support. We recommend dopamine 2–10 mg/kg/min, at which dose glomerular filtration, renal perfusion, and urine output are all increased. Poorly monitored pressor agents may result in severe vasoconstriction and end-organ ischemia.
- Heparin 20,000–30,000 U is administered IV just prior to aortic cannulation.
- After occlusion of the proximal aorta and the start of the *in situ* flush, all supportive measures may be terminated except ventilation in those cases that include lung procurements, as directed by the lung teams.

13.2. MANAGEMENT OF THE LIVER TRANSPLANT RECIPIENT

13.2.1. Preoperative Evaluation

Evaluation of the prospective liver transplant patient should include an airway evaluation, review of systems, physical examination, past surgical and anesthesia history, and relevant family history. Commonly encountered conditions associated with end-stage liver disease (ESLD) are listed in Table 13.2. Special emphasis is placed on the evaluation of the following:

TABLE 13.2. Preoperative Conditions That May Impact Anesthetic Management in Liver Transplantation

Coagulopathy (including thrombocytopenia and disseminated intravascular coagulation)
Associated problems of underlying cause of liver disease (e.g., alcoholism)
Encephalopathy
Hypokalemia
Hypocalcemia
Hypomagnesemia
Hyponatremia
Ascites
Pleural effusions
Pericardial effusions
Intrapulmonary shunting
Portal hypertension
Esophageal varices and bleeding
Increased volume of distribution
Renal insufficiency or failure
Hypoalbuminemia
Anemia

13.2.1.1. Cardiovascular System

Typically, cardiac output is supernormal, mixed venous oxygen saturation exceeds 80%, and systemic vascular resistance (SVR) is low. Peripheral arteriovenous shunting contributes to the low SVR. It is not unusual to have a patient with tachycardia and systemic blood pressure on the low side. The liver transplant procedure may be associated with large, rapid fluid and pressure shifts.

Many patients with ESLD have elevated pulmonary artery pressure (PAP). Often this is due to elevated cardiac output, and not to elevated pulmonary vascular resistance (PVR). Elevated PVR is associated with increased mortality, as patients may go into severe right ventricular failure and cardiac arrest upon reperfusion. Even though PAP can increase without a change in PVR because cardiac output is elevated, a mean PAP > 35 mmHg will usually contraindicate surgery in our Center. An increase in PVR may not be detected until insertion of a pulmonary artery catheter (PAC) at time of surgery.

The presence of a patent foramen ovale may be a contraindication to liver transplant, since pulmonary hypertension may occur during reperfusion of the liver, with right-to-left shunting and hypoxemia. Pericardial effusions occur in patients with ESLD but are usually hemodynamically insignificant. Hemodynamically significant tricuspid regurgitation (TR) may disqualify a patient. TR can lead to increases in CVP, which can lead to decreased liver blood flow. A prominent V wave on the CVP pressure trace suggests the possibility of TR. Transesophageal echocardiography (TEE) can confirm all these diagnoses.

13.2.1.2. Pulmonary System

The hepatopulmonary syndrome consists of hypoxemia due to intrapulmonary shunts. In general, this syndrome can only be cured by hepatic transplantation. Pleural effusions may compromise oxygenation during the transplant procedure. If large enough to compromise lung expansion, the effusions should be drained prior to surgery or at the time of the transplant.

13.2.1.3. Hepatorenal Syndrome

The hepatorenal syndrome is, briefly, renal failure secondary to liver disease. While the mechanisms of this syndrome are beyond the scope of this chapter, suffice it to say that hepatic transplantation is the only cure. If renal failure is severe, dialysis may be necessary prior to transplantation. Further dialysis may be needed temporarily at the conclusion of the procedure.

13.2.1.4. Metabolic System

Metabolic derangements may be multitudinous and severe. Electrolytes may be abnormal for many reasons, such as fluid overload, and cardiac and renal dysfunction. Hyponatremia is quite common, and rapid correction of significant hyponatremia should be avoided as it can lead to central pontine myelinolysis (CPM). Potassium concentrations may be either elevated or depressed depending on renal dysfunction and types of diuretics used. Mild hypocalcemia is common and usually of little clinical concern. However, if there is significant blood transfusion, calcium therapy may be required to maintain hemodynamic stability, since the diseased liver may not be capable of clearing the preservative citrate, which binds calcium, from the banked blood. Blood glucose concentrations are usually normal to elevated, depending on the presence of diabetes, and the patient's diet and hepatic function. Hypoglycemia may be seen in cases of fulminant hepatitis. Many patients arrive in the operating room with a slight metabolic acidemia, due to the accumulation of acidic metabolites not removed by the liver, or renal and circulatory dysfunction. ESLD patients may also hyperventilate, which causes respiratory alkalosis.

13.2.1.5. Neurologic System

Many patients have a mild degree of encephalopathy, which is of little concern. Severe encephalopathy places patients at risk for aspiration due to depression of protective airway reflexes. In severe liver failure, especially fulminant hepatic failure, patients are at risk for cerebral edema and elevated intracranial pressure (ICP). ICP monitoring and treatment may be necessary preoperatively to avoid irreversible neurologic injury. Intraoperatively, ICP monitoring should be continued. Arterial pressure must be maintained to provide an adequate cerebral perfusion pressure gradient ≥ 40 mmHg.

13.2.1.6. Coagulation

Thrombocytopenia is often present in patients with hypersplenism secondary to portal hypertension. This may be worsened by platelet consumption if bleeding has occurred. Fibrinogen concentrations may be low due to decreased synthesis by the diseased liver. Consumption of fibrinogen may occur appropriately during bleeding or inappropriately, if there is fibrinolysis. Other factors may be low due to decreased synthesis and/or increased consumption. It is common for the prothrombin time to be significantly elevated.

13.2.2. Perioperative Management

The general provisions for hypnosis, amnesia, analgesia, neuromuscular blockade, and hemodynamic stability must be accomplished.

13.2.2.1. General Measures

All patients are considered to be at risk for aspiration of gastric contents due to the presence of ascites, upper gastrointestinal (GI) bleeding, encephalopathy, and the nonelective scheduling. Most patients are not premedicated with sedatives. A rapid sequence induction with cricoid pressure is used. Unless contraindicated, succinylcholine is used, since a prolonged block is not a concern. If the patient is a difficult intubation, an awake oral intubation is performed. Nasal intubation is avoided because of the potential for severe epistaxis and the concern of sinus infection in an immunocompromised patient who may have a prolonged intubation. Isoflurane in air plus narcotic is the usual anesthetic technique, as this minimizes depression of splanchnic blood flow. Long-acting drugs such as pancuronium, lorazepam, and methadone may be used. Nitrous oxide is not used, in order to avoid enteric distension and enlargement of air emboli. Inspiratory oxygen concentration is maintained at 50% or less in order to avoid oxygen toxicity. Regional anesthesia for postoperative analgesia is contraindicated because of actual or potential coagulopathies.

In addition to the basic standard monitors, arterial and pulmonary artery catheters are placed. Transesophageal echocardiography may be indicated if questions arise concerning cardiac structure or function, or to detect significant pulmonary emboli. An oral gastric tube is inserted. At the end of the case, when coagulation is normalized, the oral tube can be changed to a nasal tube, and/or a feeding tube can be inserted if indicated. In our experience, esophageal instrumentation does not trigger esophageal variceal bleeding. The procedure is performed with the patient supine and arms extended. The table should have a gel pad to prevent skin damage, and intermittent pneumatic calf compression is used to prevent deep vein thrombosis and pulmonary emboli.

13.2.2.2. Hemodynamics, Lines, and Venovenous Bypass

The following monitoring lines and devices are routinely used: arterial line, usually radial or brachial; pulmonary artery catheter (PAC), via either the left internal jugular (IJ) or left subclavian vein, inserted before right IJ cannulation in order to rule out pulmonary hypertension; and the Rapid Infusor System (RIS; Haemonetics Corporation, Braintree, MA), a device that can warm and pump the contents of a reservoir at rates up to 1.5 L per minute. Large bore venous access is needed in order to permit high infusion flow rates. Packed red blood cells (PRBC), fresh-frozen plasma (FFP), and crystalloid solution are administered via the RIS. If the patient starts with a high hematocrit, only crystalloid and/or FFP is added until the patient's hematocrit dilutes down to approximately 28%. At this point, FFP, PRBC, and crystalloid solution are added to the reservoir as needed in the ratio of 1 unit PRBC:1 unit FFP:250 ml crystalloid. Platelets and cryoprecipitate are not administered via the RIS.

Venovenous bypass is used to divert inferior vena cava and portal blood flow around the retrohepatic portion of the inferior vena cava when it is clamped. One cannula, therefore, must be placed distal to the clamped portion (i.e., in the femoral artery) and the other in a tributary of the superior vena cava (i.e., right IJ or axillary vein). A third cannula is inserted intraoperatively by the surgeon into the recipient's native portal vein, thus permitting the portal blood flow to join the return from the femoral vein en route to the centrifugal bypass pump. The traditional method of intraoperative surgical cutdown of the femoral and axillary veins adds to surgical time and leaves the patient with two additional incisions and potential associated complications. Alternately and preferably, percutaneous insertion of two 16 French cannulae, one in a femoral vein and the other in the right IJ vein, is used. The right IJ cannula also serves as the infusion site for the RIS. If the right IJ cannot be cannulated, the surgeon will need to do an axillary vein cutdown. If bypass is not a requirement of the surgical procedure, then these cannulae are not needed. Minimum infusion rates of 50 cc/hour through both cannulae should be maintained throughout the operation in order to prevent clotting.

Inotropes, vasoconstrictors, calcium chloride, and nitroglycerin should be immediately available. Epinephrine, norepinephrine, and phenylephrine are the agents most commonly used at our Center. Nitroglycerin is occasionally needed after reperfusion if pulmonary artery pressures are elevated. Transfusion of blood components is often necessary during liver transplantation. PRBC and FFP are administered via the RIS. Platelets and cryoprecipitate are generally administered via a peripheral or central vein after proper filtration. Due to the possibility of ventricular fibrillation during reperfusion of the donor liver, adhesive defibrillation pads are placed on the chest prior to prep and drape. This facilitates rapid defibrillation should the need arise.

13.2.2.3. Antibiotics, Immunosuppression, and Cytoprotection

An antibiotic (3 g Unasyn® in non-penicillin-allergic patients) and methylprednisolone (50 mg) are given prior to incision. Following anastomosis of the hepatic artery, Unasyn® (1.5 g) and methylprednisolone (1 g) are administered. Prostaglandin E1 (PGE1) is administered at a rate of 0.3–0.6 µg/kg/hr in the postanhepatic portion of the surgery as a hepatic and renal cytoprotective agent. PGE1 is a potent arterial and pulmonary vasodilator and may need to be decreased or discontinued if it causes unacceptable hypotension.

13.2.2.4. Temperature Management

Maintenance of temperature is important for general homeostasis but particularly for optimization of the coagulation system. Room temperature is a critical determinant of heat loss, so the room should be warm enough to minimize heat loss. Other methods include the use of warm air blankets, fluid warming via the RIS, low fresh gas flow rates, and heat–moisture exchangers. If the venovenous bypass circuit is used, a heating element may be placed in-line.

13.2.3. Intraoperative Management

The surgical procedure can be divided into four sequential time periods: hepatectomy, anhepatic, reperfusion, and postreperfusion.

During the hepatectomy, the liver is dissected and prepared for removal. There is a potential for massive hemorrhage because of preexisting coagulopathy, portal hypertension, and potentially difficult surgical dissection. Laboratory (prothrombin time [OT], partial thromboplastin time [PTT], fibrinogen, and platelet count) and/or thromboelastography results guide replacement of factors and platelets. An attempt to normalize coagulation should be made prior to institution of venovenous bypass. Hemodynamic instability can be due to hemorrhage as well as retraction on the inferior vena cava, both of which can decrease preload. Replacement fluids are guided by PAC trends, urine output, and blood loss.

The acid–base status is generally near normal, although critically ill patients may have a metabolic acidemia. Mild acidemia is often not treated. However, if hemodynamics are unstable or the acidemia worsens, treatment is initiated with sodium bicarbonate. In cases where there is significant hyponatremia and adequate renal function, tromethamine (THAM) is used as an alternative to sodium bicarbonate. About one-third as potent as sodium bicarbonate, THAM is a potassium salt. Careful, serial potassium measurements should be made when using THAM.

Hypocalcemia is often a problem during rapid transfusions due to the citrate in banked blood products. Hypotension is often the result and may be quickly treated with small amounts of calcium chloride. A more difficult situation may occur after the hepatic artery is ligated. The ischemic liver may accumulate calcium ions to the point that symptomatic hypocalcemia occurs. Observation of the QT interval on the electrocardiogram (EKG) may provide evidence that this is occurring. Measurement confirms the diagnosis and treatment is symptomatic and is needed only until the ischemic liver is removed.

Blood glucose levels may be elevated in diabetics, in which case an insulin infusion may be necessary. Once the incision is made, hypoglycemia is generally not a problem due to catecholamine-induced glycogenolysis. Cachectic patients with long-standing poor nutrition may be hypoglycemic and not respond to sympathetic outflow if glycogen stores are minimal. Small amounts of glucose are generally sufficient to maintain blood glucose levels near normal.

Renal dysfunction is common in patients undergoing liver transplant. The hepatorenal syndrome increases creatinine and reduces urine flow. Renal venous hypertension during manipulation of the inferior vena cava may temporarily decrease urine output. Urine output generally improves after the new liver is reperfused. If blood pressure permits, infusions of PGE1 may improve renal blood flow and urine output. Dopamine infusions have also been used.

Venovenous bypass (VVB) is designed to reroute inferior vena cava and portal blood around the clamped and resected liver and intrahepatic cava, and returns blood to the heart. It is thus two-limbed (i.e., femoral and portal veins) on the inflow side of the pump and single-limbed as it return blood to the superior vena cava. It helps maintain cardiac preload while at the same time avoiding engorgement of splanchnic, renal, and lower extremity venous systems. Techniques of liver transplantation that do not require complete clamping of the inferior vena cava, the "piggyback" technique, may not require VVB, since inferior vena caval flow is not interrupted. VVB is indicated in patients with a history of GI bleeding, significant portal hypertension, difficult liver dissections, renal insufficiency, borderline cardiac function, and hemodynamic instability during a 10-minute test clamping of the inferior vena cava. Complications may be divided into those associated with venous cannulation and the circuit itself. Cannulation-related complications include venous injury, infection, and/or seroma formation. The bypass circuit may produce traumatic injury to cellular elements of blood as well as the activation and perhaps consumption of platelets. Flow rates below 1 L/min have been associated with thrombus formation and pulmonary emboli. Despite these potential problems, VVB is generally very well tolerated.

The anhepatic phase encompasses the time when the recipient liver has been removed and the donor liver is reperfused. During this phase, worsening metabolic acidemia and hypocalcemia develop. These should be treated prior to reperfusion. Hypokalemia is generally not treated unless symptomatic, because reperfusion of the liver generally causes the potassium concentration to rise. Coagulopathies may worsen, and appropriate replacement therapy is ordered. Platelets and cryoprecipitate are generally not given until the postbypass period to avoid clotting of the circuit. Decreased urine output may occur whether bypass is used or not. If blood pressure permits, PGE1 is either initiated or continued.

The sequence of anastomoses is as follows: suprahepatic cava, infrahepatic cava, portal vein, hepatic artery, and biliary. Prior to completion of the infrahepatic cava anastomosis, one liter of iced Ringer's lactate is infused under 300 mmHg pressure into the donor portal vein in order to flush out the preservation solution. This simple maneuver has significantly decreased the severity of reperfusion reactions. In order to anastomose the portal vein, one limb of the VVB is removed. This may decrease preload significantly and lead to hypotension. Small amounts of vasoconstrictors may be needed at this time. Volume infusion is withheld unless absolutely needed, because a significant increase in preload usually occurs during unclamping and reperfusion.

The liver is reperfused when the portal vein is unclamped and the inferior vena cava is opened. Hypotension commonly occurs when the liver is reperfused and is most likely to occur in livers with long ischemic times. Dysrhythmias secondary to hyperkalemia may further complicate matters. In the absence of rhythm disturbances, small amounts of calcium and epinephrine are usually efficacious. The hypotension is generally short-lived and requires only symptomatic treatment. Transient pulmonary hypertension may be due to vasoconstrictive substances released from an ischemic liver, air or thrombotic emboli, or myocardial depression. If the systemic pressure is adequate, it may not need treatment. This elevated PAP usually normalizes over a variable period of time (minutes to hours). A reoccurrence of elevated PAP implies another process (i.e., pulmonary embolism) is occurring that requires evaluation and treatment if indicated. Elevated CVP may also occur and compromise hepatic blood flow. If this occurs, nitroglycerin and/or inotropic therapy may be needed to enhance right ventricular function and decrease CVP. Discontinuation of VVB occurs after reperfusion is satisfactory and all surgical anastomoses are checked for hemostasis. Blood remaining in the bypass circuit should be reinfused if possible. Blood should not be reinfused if it will significantly elevate CVP and cause hepatic engorgement.

After reperfusion, the hepatic artery is anastomosed, if this has not been done previously. The liver is now completely perfused. With a well-functioning graft, the liver beings to synthesize coagulation factors, and both coagulation and the overall clinical situation begin to improve. A well-functioning graft produces bile, and looks and feels appropriate, with normal color and texture, and has sharp edges. (A hard and red liver may reflect an inflammatory process with impedance to hepatic blood flow; rounded edges suggest an edematous process.) Urine output improves and the metabolic acidosis resolves. Metabolism of the calcium–citrate complexes may result in hypercalcemia and alkalosis. Glucose levels frequently increase. In contrast, a deterioration of the overall clinical status should prompt discussion with the surgeon, as such may reflect a poorly or nonfunctioning graft.

13.3. MANAGEMENT OF THE KIDNEY TRANSPLANT RECIPIENT

In addition to providing anesthesia for a patient with end-stage renal disease (ESRD), the goal of management includes providing the best environment for the newly implanted kidney. One must consider the implications of the underlying disease that caused the ESRD (e.g., diabetes and hypertension), as well as the effect of ESRD on other organ systems (Table 13.3).

General anesthesia is usually employed. Although region anesthesia has been used for kidney transplant, many patients have some degree of coagulopathy, and hemodynamic management may be difficult given the unknown status of intravascular volume and autonomic neuropathy.

With long preservation times, patients may have had the opportunity to fast for > 8 hours, but may have other issues that make them candidates for rapid sequence (delayed gastric emptying, increased gastric volume and acidity). Patients should be dialyzed prior to transplant. Succinylcholine can be used if the serum potassium level is ≤ 5.5 mEq/L.

The induction agents etomidate, benzodiazepine, barbiturate, and/or ketamine can all be used and are metabolized mainly by liver. While an increased cardiac output would suggest need for a higher dose of induction agent, decreased protein binding and a less than fully intact blood–brain barrier would suggest a need for less. In practice, these factors tend to negate each other, and the dose of induction agent is determined by factors other than just having renal disease.

It is not uncommon to get a large swing in blood pressure secondary to inadequate compensation due to autonomic neuropathy and the effect of antihypertensive medications that the patient may be taking.

Anesthesia is usually maintained with nitrous oxide, oxygen, isoflurane, and opioid narcotics. Enflurane is avoided because of the potential nephrotoxic effect of fluoride. Sevoflurane is avoided because of potential nephrotoxic metabolites. Halothane is avoided because many patients with ESRD also have liver disease.

TABLE 13.3. Physiological Derangements in ESRD Patients

Chronic anemia—decreased production and decreased survival	Central and peripheral nervous system
	Lethargy to coma
Increased cardiac output	Dementia
Oxyhemoglobin dissociation curve shifted to the right	Aluminum toxicity from dialysate or antacids
Coagulopathies	Seizures
Platelet dysfunction	Uremia
Systemic heparinization (after dialysis)	Hypertension
Altered hydration	Peripheral neuropathies
Unpredictable intravascular fluid (before or in need of dialysis)	Autonomic neuropathy
	Gastrointestinal
Electrolyte imbalance	Increased gastric fluid and acidity
Hyperkalemia	Delayed gastric emptying
Hypermagnesemia	Nausea and vomiting
Hypocalcemia	Endocrine dysfunction
Hyperphosphatemia	Hyperparathyroidism leading to osteodystrophy
Metabolic acidosis	
Cardiovascular	Glucose intolerance
Systemic hypertension	Pancreatitis
Congestive heart failure	Musculoskeletal
Pericarditis	Renal osteodystrophy
Dysrhythmias (abnormal electrolytes)	Generalized muscle weakness
Pulmonary	Metastatic calcification
Pleural effusions	Gout and pseudogout
Pulmonary edema	Integument
Immunocompromised	Pruritis
Decreased activity of phagocytes	Hyperpigmentation
Immunosuppressant medications	

Muscle relaxation is usually accomplished with either cisatracurium or atracurium, as neither medication depends on the kidneys for elimination. The antagonist neostigmine is 50% renally excreted; therefore, there may be a prolonged effect.

Many of these patients have either an arteriovenous (AV) graft or fistula for hemodialysis access. These must be protected, as they may still be needed postoperatively in case of graft nonfunction. No intravenous or blood pressure cuff should be placed on the extremity with the access site.

After Foley catheter insertion, fluid is instilled to distend the bladder, in order to facilitate surgical ureter–bladder anastomosis. The clamp on the Foley should not be removed until the surgical team requests it. Therefore, there is no monitor of urine output until late in the case. However, many of these patients are anuric or oliguric because of their underlying ESRD.

A CVP line is used in all patients. Posttransplant renal failure can result from prerenal, renal, or postrenal causes. Adequate hydration with potassium-free fluid guided by CVP monitoring tends to minimize the possibility of prerenal failure. The protocol at our Center is to maintain a CVP of 10–12 cm water. On rare occasions, a patient will go into pulmonary edema, particularly if there is nonfunction of the graft.

Mannitol, 25 g, and furosemide, 100 mg, are administered when the transplanted kidney is exposed to recipient circulation. Initial urine output after clamp removal reflects prior fluid instillation into the bladder. Fifteen minutes after clamp removal, output from the Foley catheter is then assumed to represent kidney production.

Many ESRD patients are diabetics. Glucose monitoring and control may be needed. Strict aseptic technique for line placement should be used in these immunocompromised patients. Although kidney transplants are usually performed with little blood loss, these patients are often anemic, and transfusion may be needed if significant blood loss occurs.

Although there is usually no or very little systemic effect, cardiac arrest after completion of renal artery anastomosis has been reported, most likely due to the release of potassium from the preservation solution to the general circulation. Additionally, clamping of the external iliac artery may be necessary during renal artery anastomosis. The release of this clamp is usually not associated with any significant systemic effect, but in theory, reperfusion problems (e.g., hypotension secondary to fluid shifts) can occur.

Rapid acute immunologic rejection can occur, which probably reflects prior sensitization to specific donor antigens. Inadequate circulation to new kidney may be evident on the surgical field. Delayed signs may present with hyperthermia, deterioration of urine output, and disseminated intravascular coagulation (DIC). If detected, these signs should be reported to the surgical team.

Postoperatively, excessive hypertension should be avoided in order to protect the vascular anastomosis. Hypotension can lead to inadequate perfusion to the new kidney and access graft. Finally, although the recipient needs to be adequately volume loaded in order to avoid prerenal failure, if the new kidney does not work or is delayed in functioning, fluid overload and pulmonary edema may result.

13.4. MANAGEMENT OF THE PANCREAS TRANSPLANT RECIPIENT

Since a pancreas transplant is generally performed in combination with a renal transplant, this section focuses on the pancreas transplant, because the kidney transplant-recipient discussion also applies during the combined transplant.

Pancreas transplants are performed in patients with severe diabetes mellitus. These patients often have peripheral and autonomic neuropathies. Atherosclerosis is frequent and puts these patients at risk for coronary artery disease, cardiomyopathy, cerebral vascular accidents, and peripheral vascular disease. These patients are immunocompromised, because they suffer from leukocyte dysfunction.

The major additional task in these surgical patients is to manage glucose levels. Hypoglycemia must be avoided, as it can lead to brain damage. Similarly, uncontrolled hyperglycemia can lead to dehydration and electrolyte disturbances. Ketoacidosis can also occur and should be avoided.

Since the signs of hypoglycemia can be masked by general anesthesia, blood, not urine, glucose levels need to be measured. Glucose levels should be checked 30–60 minutes after insulin administration and every hour, for 4 hours. After the pancreas is in, glucose levels should be monitored every 20 minutes, as there may be excess insulin production. Dextrose infusion or ampule administration may be needed, as hypoglycemia may otherwise occur.

Part IV

Immediate Postoperative Care and Complications

Chapter 14

Postoperative Care in Liver Transplantation

Jorge A. Ortiz

The liver transplant recipient shares many issues with the critical general or vascular surgery patient. As an example, continued hemorrhage, intestinal perforation, atelectasis, and pulmonary embolism are treated similarly. However, because of immunosuppression and a host of other factors, the liver transplant recipient's management can become very complicated. Fluid shifts, viral and fungal infections, graft nonfunction, and rejection are examples of issues unique to the transplant patient. The following is a systems approach to the critically ill postoperative liver transplant recipient.

14.1. GENERAL INTENSIVE CARE ISSUES

After the liver transplant procedure is completed, the patient is transferred to the intensive care unit (ICU) in guarded condition. Rarely, the patient is extubated on the operating room table. Most often however, *ventilator support* is necessary for 24–48 hours. Those with extended ventilator dependence have a significantly increased mortality. A number of respiratory and metabolic issues may manifest themselves during this critical period. Oversedation or early graft dysfunction may precipitate hypercarbic *respiratory acidosis*. The treatment is withdrawal of sedatives and pain medications. A deranged mental status that leads to hypercarbia may be a sign of early graft dysfunction and consideration should be given to retransplantation. *Metabolic alkalosis* may result from metabolism of the blood products given in the operating room combined with aggressive diuresis and hypokalemia. Judicious administration of potassium is necessary to replenish intracellular stores. Some centers give hydrochloric acid in order to combat the metabolic alkalosis. Regardless, metabolic and respiratory acid–base derangements usually correct within 48 hours with prudent electrolyte administration, ventilator management, and a properly functioning liver.

Hypoxia in the early postoperative period may result from a number of factors, including hepatopulmonary syndrome, atelectasis, pleural effusions, central nervous system depression, pulmonary edema, pulmonary embolus, pneumonia, pneumonitis, and acute respiratory distress syndrome (ARDS). Hepatopulmonary syndrome improves over weeks to months after liver transplantation. Not infrequently, the patient requires supplemental oxygen therapy in the ICU and for many months postoperatively. *Atelectasis* commonly occurs after major abdominal surgery. The presence of ascites, diaphragmatic dysfunction, decreased lung compliance, and poor respiratory effort may conspire to worsen pulmonary function. Chest physiotherapy and positive pressure ventilation are frequently necessary in order to expand collapsed alveoli and improve ventilation. Up to 20% of patients may require therapeutic bronchoscopy.

Pleural effusions are common and usually occur on the right side. They are transudative in nature. Those that cause respiratory embarrassment and do not respond to aggressive diuresis may need therapeutic drainage. Large bore chest tubes are avoided in the early postoperative period because of the risk of life-threatening hemorrhage. Smaller "pigtail" catheters can be safely placed in the pleural cavity, with or without ultrasound guidance. It is important to note that the diaphragm is frequently elevated postoperatively, which increases the chance of intra-abdominal placement of catheters meant for the thoracic cavity. Generally, pleural effusions resolve within 1 to 2 weeks after surgery.

A poorly functioning graft and/or overadministration of narcotics and sedatives may cause *central nervous system depression* and hypoxia. Close attention must be paid to proper dosing schedules of various medications. A patient with continued mental status changes, coagulopathy, hemodynamic instability, and rising liver function tests should be considered for retransplantation.

Patients with *pulmonary edema* will have crackles and wheezes on auscultation, increased peripheral and sacral swelling, increased pulmonary capillary wedge pressures, and chest roentgenographic examinations consistent with fluid overload. Snowden et al. (*Liver Transplantation* 2000;6,4:466–470) reported an incidence of pulmonary edema in 47% of orthotopic liver transplantation (OLT) recipients after surgery. Patients with higher transfusion requirements had a greater likelihood of showing deterioration of gaseous exchange and other clinical effects consistent with this diagnosis. If renal function is adequate, patients will respond to diuresis. At times, respiratory compromise is so severe that temporary reintubation may be necessary. Patients with renal failure may need dialysis or hemofiltration. Pulmonary edema may result from excessive hydration, but it may also be a manifestation of cardiac failure. Therefore, electrocardiograms (EKGs), cardiac enzymes, and possibly echocardiographs should be evaluated to rule out cardiogenic pulmonary edema.

Pulmonary emboli are rare after transplantation because of abnormal clotting in the immediate postoperative period. Administration of clotting factors and bedrest may increase the risk. Hypercoagulable states, such as those seen with Budd–Chiari syndrome, place patients in jeopardy of emboli formation. Those patients identified with a hypercoagulable state should be anticoagulated postoperatively. If a patient is hypoxemic with tachycardia, ventilation/perfusion mismatching, and an increased alveolar-arterial gradient, the diagnosis of pulmonary embolism should be seriously considered. Heparinization and even pulmonary embolectomy may be necessary after the diagnosis is confirmed.

Acute respiratory distress syndrome (ARDS) may occur immediately or up to several weeks postoperatively. The reported incidence varies from 5% to 15%. Precipitating factors include the sepsis syndrome, pneumonitis and OKT3 (a drug for acute organ rejection) administration. ARDS is diagnosed in the hypoxic patient with ground-glass appearance on chest X-ray, decreased pulmonary compliance, and low or normal pulmonary capillary filling pressures. The treatment is correction of the inciting causes, antibiotics for sepsis, appropriate drainage of collections, ventilatory support, and judicious management of fluids.

Pneumonitis may result from aspiration of blood or gastric contents. The treatment is, once again, supportive. Antibiotics may be employed to protect against pneumonia. Ventilator support is frequently necessary. Nursing precautions such as elevation of the head of the bed, tube feeding while awake, and ensuring properly functioning nasogastric tubes are paramount if one is to avoid this potentially fatal complication.

Pneumonia is the most common pulmonary complication. Early on, it is usually bacterial in origin. However fungal and viral pneumonias are not uncommon. Proper prophylaxis entails the use of perioperative antibiotics, antiviral medications, antifungal medications when appropriate, and sulfa derivatives to prevent *Pneumocystis carinii.* The diagnosis is made in the febrile transplant recipient with positive sputum cultures or lavage and/or an abnormal infiltrate on chest X-ray. Treatment is directed at the isolated organism.

Extended *ventilator dependence* may result from any of the aforementioned causes. Additionally, preoperative malnutrition and deconditioning may lead to an inability to extubate. Proper nursing care and nutritional support via the enteral and parenteral routes are paramount for postsurgical rehabilitation.

14.2. RENAL DYSFUNCTION

Not uncommon after liver transplantation, renal dysfunction may result from acute tubular necrosis (ATN), drug toxicity, hypovolemia, abdominal compartment syndrome, and hepatorenal syndrome. *Risk factors* include intraoperative hypotension, allograft dysfunction, and preoperative hepatorenal syndrome. Oliguria is the earliest sign of dysfunction. Subsequent blood urea nitrogen (BUN) and creatinine elevations confirm the diagnosis. The hypovolemic patient will respond to hydration. The *indications for dialysis* are the same as in the nontransplant patient, that is, acidosis, hyperkalemia, fluid overload, and uremic pericarditis. In patients who are fluid overloaded yet too unstable to tolerate conventional dialysis, *continuous venovenous hemofiltration* may be beneficial. ATN and hepatorenal syndrome are frequently self-limiting and may respond to prudent diuretic administration. *Abdominal compartment syndrome* is usually seen in the fluid-overloaded patient with a tight, distended abdomen. Paracentesis or reexploration and open packing of the wound may be necessary. The doses of potentially *nephrotoxic medications* such as Gentamycin, calcineurin inhibitors, angiotensin-converting enzyme (ACE) inhibitors, and H2-blockers should all be adjusted appropriately. In the majority of patients, postoperative renal dysfunction resolves without the need for chronic dialysis.

14.3. NEUROLOGIC ISSUES

Neurologic complications occur in 12–20% of patients after liver transplantation. Eighty-five percent of these complications occur in the first postoperative week. The symptoms and signs range from seizures to disorientation, to agitation, to coma, and are more likely in older patients and those with severe encephalopathy preoperatively. The *causes* include "toxic-metabolic" processes, hypomagnesemia, hypoglycemia, hypercalcemia, hypo- and hypernatremia (central pontine myelinolysis), poor graft function, drug reactions, infections, and intracranial hemorrhage. *Medications* should be carefully reviewed in order to identify agents that may be the cause of the neurologic changes. These include amantadine, cyclosporine, steroids, narcotic analgesics, histamine type 2 blockers, acyclovir, antibiotics (e.g., Imipenem), benzodiazepines, and tacrolimus. There should be a low threshold for obtaining blood, urine, and sputum cultures, and a computerized tomographic (CT) scan of the head and an electroencephalogram (EEG). An EEG may reveal subclinical seizure activity. A CT scan may show intracranial bleeds, multiple infarcts, or abscesses. Those at risk for bleeds include patients who are hemodynamically unstable, with massive transfusion requirements and coagulopathy. *Neurosurgical maneuvers* are required if there is midline shift or evidence of increased intracranial pressure. The mortality for intracranial bleeds after liver transplantation may be as high as 80%.

14.4. CARDIOVASCULAR ISSUES

Hypertension after transplantation is seen in 50–75% of patients in the first weeks and months following surgery. Frequently a patient's essential hypertension is unmasked by correction of his or her hyperdynamic state and worsened by the administration of tacrolimus or cyclosporine. Tacrolimus causes less hypertension than cyclosporine. The additive effect of corticosteroids and calcineurin inhibitors in the exacerbation of hypertension mandates reduction in immunosuppression whenever clinically feasible. Arterial pressure elevations result from increased systemic vascular resistance based on vasoconstriction. Prudent administration of beta and calcium channel blockers usually suffices to correct the hypertension. ACE inhibitors are not recommended in the early postoperative period because renin levels are low at this point. It is important to note that hypertension (and tachycardia) can result from renal dose dopamine.

Hypotension results from falling behind in the resuscitation efforts with intravenous fluids and or blood products. Continued hypotension and transfusion requirements mandate consideration for reexploration. Use of prostaglandin E1 (PGE1) frequently causes hypotension as well.

Tachycardia may be caused by inadequate pain control, hypovolemia, pulmonary embolus, and dopamine administration.

Bradycardia may result from sick sinus syndrome, infections, overdosage of antiarrhythmics and antihypertensives, and increased intracranial pressures.

Cardiac failure accounts for a 7–21% mortality rate after liver transplantation. Therefore, recognition and proper treatment of cirrhotic cardiomyopathy are essential. Such dysfunction can occur independent of prior alcohol abuse. It may be missed by standard echocardiographic techniques. The liver transplantation procedure, with its attendant hemodynamic and volume shifts, stresses the heart significantly. Acid–base abnormalities, hypothermia, and electrolyte disturbances can also affect myocardial function. As the hyperdynamic physiology of cirrhosis is corrected postprocedure, vasoconstriction causes increased afterload and may precipitate heart failure. Management strategies include diuretics, salt restriction, afterload reduction, and possibly mechanical ventilation. Cirrhotic cardiomyopathy may improve after liver transplant.

14.5. HEMATOLOGIC ALTERATIONS

Liver transplant recipients may suffer a number of hematologic adverse events in the immediate postoperative period. Anemia, thrombocytopenia, and neutropenia may result from surgical, infectious, and pharmacologic causes.

Anemia may be dilutional as a result of overaggressive administration of intravenous fluids or inadequate replacement of blood products in the operating room. Continued surgical bleeding occurs in 7–15% of cases and results in reexploration in half of those cases. Other causes of bleeding include ulcers, viral enteritis, portal hypertensive lesions, and Roux-en-Y bleeds. Therefore, aggressive diagnostic and therapeutic maneuvers are crucial in the early postoperative period. These include upper and lower endoscopy, bleeding scans, angiograms, and reexploration. It is imperative that medical coagulopathy be corrected judiciously. Ulcer prophylaxis is usually adequate with proton pump inhibitors. Variceal bleeds may result from a thrombosed hepatic artery or portal vein.

If the hemoglobin is too high (particularly in pediatric patients), therapeutic *phlebotomy* may be necessary to prevent vascular thrombosis.

Thrombocytopenia may result from continued splenic sequestration, drug toxicity (furosemide, mycophenolate), infections (herpes, parvovirus, sepsis syndrome), preformed antibodies, and rejection. Usually it is safe to allow a platelet count of 20,000 as long as there is no bleeding. With a well-functioning graft, thrombocytopenia should resolve within 1 week.

Neutropenia may result from drug toxicity (mycophenolate and rapamycin) and infections as well. The treatment is aimed at the inciting agent. Neupogen® is sometimes given when the counts are low.

Elevated white blood cell counts usually signal ongoing infection but may just reflect steroid effect.

Coagulopathy seen in the cirrhotic frequently persists postoperatively. If the patient is not bleeding and/or the prothrombin time (PT) is ≤ 22 seconds, cautious observation is recommended. In the face of bleeding or higher PT, prudent administration of factors such as fresh-frozen plasma and cryoprecipitate (if the fibrinogen is lower than 100) may be necessary.

14.6. INFECTIONS IN THE IMMEDIATE POSTOPERATIVE PERIOD

Mortality related to infection in liver transplant recipients is 10%. Because of immunosuppression, anergy, and malnutrition, infected liver transplant patients do not present with classic findings. Not infrequently a recipient may be infected and not demonstrate an elevated white blood cell (WBC) count or fever. In a recent study, 23% of all infections were unaccompanied by fever and 9% were accompanied by hypothermia. Bile peritonitis may be present in a patient with a soft, nontender abdomen. It is therefore imperative to have a *high index of suspicion*. A pulmonary infiltrate, with or without fever or elevated WBC, is likely to be pneumonia. Greenish output from an abdominal drain is bile peritonitis until proven otherwise, regardless of temperature or physical examination. Additionally, those patients who do have fever in the ICU are very likely (87%) to have infection. In the ICU, 79% of infections are bacterial, 9% viral, and 9% fungal. In all liver transplant recipients, 55% of infections are bacterial, 22% fungal, and 22% viral. Over half of *bacterial infections* occur in the first two postoperative weeks, which is the time of greatest immunosuppression. The etiology of most bacterial infections is usually Gram-positive bacteria. Treatment is based on isolation of the offending organism, surgical or percutaneous drainage when appropriate, and proper antibiotic coverage. Risk factors for bacterial infection are extremes of age, malnutrition, prolonged hospital stay, prolonged operative time, increased blood transfusions, and surgical complications such as hepatic artery thrombosis and biliary obstruction or leak. Prophylaxis is targeted at Gram-positive organisms such as staphylococcal and enteric bacteria. Ampicillin or Piperacillin are frequently employed for 2–7 days postoperatively. In penicillin-allergic patients, Vancomycin is frequently used with a second- or third-generation cephalosporin.

Fungal infections occur most commonly in the first 8 weeks after transplantation. Risk factors are similar to those for bacterial infection. Candida is the most frequent culprit. Treatment is with amphotericin or its liposomal formulations, or fluconazole. Prophylaxis in high-risk patients may be warranted. However, excessive use of fluconazole prophylaxis has led to the emergence of resistant strains. Aspergillus accounts for approximately 15% of all fungal infections and is responsible for 90% of brain abscesses. Treatment is with amphotericin and/or itraconazole. There are studies evaluating the utility of itraconazole prophylaxis. No benefit has been shown.

Pneumocystis carinii is a parasite infection that usually affects patients late after transplantation. Prophylaxis is with trimethoprim–sulfamethoxazole. Data support its use for at least 1 year.

Most *viral infections* occur between 3 and 4 weeks postoperatively. However, up to 10% of infections in the immediate postoperative period are viral in nature. Reactivation of cytomegalovirus (CMV) is a major cause of viral infection. CMV syndrome is manifested by fever, myalgia, malaise, leukopenia, and thrombocytopenia. The liver allograft is the most common site of organ involvement. Treatment and prophylaxis with immune globulin preparations, gancyclovir (IV and by mouth), and/or acyclovir are extremely effective. This regimen should last approximately 100 days.

14.7. PRIMARY GRAFT NONFUNCTION (PNF)

PNF is the most common cause of graft loss in the immediate postoperative period. It is generally defined as immediate perioperative graft failure with coagulopathy, acidosis, hypothermia, encephalopathy, decreased bile output, and elevated liver function tests. The incidence ranges between 2% and 10%. The *risk factors* include, but are not limited to, advanced donor age, steatosis, and prolonged cold and warm ischemia time. Ischemia–reperfusion injury, free radical production, leukotrienes, thromboxanes, other immune-mediated events, and possible metabolic derangements, all may play a role in its pathogenesis. Early PNF may improve with supportive care or with the administration of PGE1. Unfortunately, *retransplantation* is the only option for patients who remain encephalopathic, acidotic, hypoglycemic, hypothermic, and coagulopathic. A liver biopsy with greater than 50% necrosis confirms the diagnosis but is unreliable and rarely performed. If a liver does not become available, hepatectomy with portocaval shunting or continuous bypass may become necessary until a proper donor is identified.

14.8. HEMORRHAGIC NECROSIS

The Miami group (*Transplantation* 1996;*61*,9:1370–1376) has described the following scenario: Following rejection and allograft dysfunction, fever and massive graft failure ensue in the absence of vascular thrombosis. The only treatment is believed to be retransplantation.

14.9. INDUCTION IMMUNOSUPPRESSION

Although graft loss from rejection has decreased to the 5% range in the cyclosporine/tacrolimus era, it continues to affect up to 100% of recipients in the first year. Therefore, the concept of induction therapy in order to reduce perioperative rejection and possibly improve long-term allograft function is particularly attractive. Those medications employed for perioperative induction include poly- and monoclonal antibodies, interleukin 2 receptor (IL-2R) antagonists, and mycophenolate mofetil. Antithymocyte globulins (ATGs) and OKT3 have been used with and without calcineurin inhibitors for many years. The purpose was to continue strong immunosuppression while avoiding nephrotoxicity and hepatotoxicity in the immediate recovery period. A number of studies have since been performed and the consensus among most transplant centers is to reserve ATG and OKT3 for treatment of steroid-resistant rejection. Mycophenolate and the IL-2R antogonists have superior side-effect profiles. However, to date no randomized prospective double-blind studies have been published. Anecdotal evidence may point to a slightly decreased risk of rejection with these two classes of immunosuppressants. Unfortunately, a significant number of patients are forced to switch off of mycophenolate because of gastrointestinal side effects. Therefore, at this point, induction immunosuppression cannot be recommended in the routine liver transplant recipient.

14.10. HEPATIC ARTERY

Inflow to the allograft via the hepatic artery can be compromised because of aneurysm, stenosis, disruption, and thrombosis. The incidence of *hepatic artery thrombosis* (HAT) in adults ranges from 2% to 8%. These patients can present in fulminant hepatic necrosis with bacteremia, hemodynamic instability, and markedly elevated liver enzymes. They can also demonstrate a more indolent course with relapsing bacteremia, milder elevations of liver enzymes, and hepatic abscesses on CT scans and ultrasounds. Late presentation may be primarily biliary in nature, with cholangitis and bile duct strictures. The *causes* of HAT include technical factors such as intimal dissection, kink, stenosis, clamp injury, and compression of the celiac axis by the arcuate ligament. Risk factors for HAT include CMV mismatching of donor and recipient, prolonged cold ischemia time, increased hematocrit, deficiency of protein C, protein S, and antithrombin III. Additionally, small arteries anastomosed without microscope magnification, split donors, and decreased arterial flow noted after completion of the anastomosis are technical issues that may predispose to an increased incidence of HAT.

The *diagnosis* is made on duplex scanning and angiography. A newer modality yet to be completely evaluated is spiral computerized tomography. When patients present with fulminant hepatic necrosis, the graft should be removed and a new organ transplanted. If the patient is symptomatic without fulminant hepatic failure, revascularization within 24 hours of diagnosis has proven beneficial. Patients with localized necrosis may benefit from local resection. There are patients who thrombose their artery and do not become unstable hemodynamically, nor do they develop strictures or abscesses. Some centers recommend expectant management in asymptomatic patients in the early postoperative period with a thrombosed artery. Unfortunately, in 50–70% of patients, retransplantation is necessary.

Hepatic artery stenosis usually presents with an insidious decrease in graft function or the onset of biliary complications. Ultrasonographic findings include resistive indices < 0.5, systolic acceleration, or increases in focal peak velocity. This can be treated with percutaneous transluminal angioplasty or rearterialization.

Hepatic artery pseudoaneurysms may present with gastrointestinal and sometimes intra-abdominal bleeding, and are diagnosed with ultrasound and angiography. They are usually involved with local (frequently fungal) infection. Treatment is resection of the involved area and revascularization. Sometimes retransplantation is necessary.

14.11. PORTAL VEIN

Portal vein thrombosis (PVT) occurs in 1–2% of patients. Risk factors include pediatric recipient, split donation, hypercoagulable states, malignancy, splenectomy, shunt surgery, and prior PVT. It may manifest with hepatic dysfunction, ascites, variceal bleeding, and hemodynamic instability. Diagnosis is made with Doppler ultrasound and confirmed with angiography. Treatment options include operative thrombectomy, retransplantation and percutaneous transluminal angioplasty, thrombolysis, and stenting. Angioplasty is performed either trans-hepatically or via the transjugular route. There is no unanimity concerning the use of aspirin or coumadin after portal vein thrombosis has been successfully treated. Rethrombosis rates are approximately 9%. *Portal vein stenosis* presents similarly and may necessitate reoperation or angioplasty.

14.12. INFERIOR VENA CAVA (IVC) AND HEPATIC VEINS

The IVC and hepatic veins become *stenosed* or *obstructed* in 1–2% of cases. These patients present with renal failure, ascites, lower extremity edema, and liver dysfunction. The diagnosis is made with ultrasound and confirmed with angiography. Symptoms usually develop if the pressure gradient is greater than 5–6 mmHg. Treatment is usually with percutaneous dilatation, with or without stenting. Sometimes reanastomosis or even retransplantation is necessary. When the conventional approach is used, the superior vena cava is more frequently affected.

14.13. BILIARY SYSTEM

Biliary complications, such as *leakage* or *obstruction*, occur in 8–15% of patients, with a mortality rate of 10%. Most occur within the first month of surgery. Changes in biliary output from the T tube (if present), biliary leakage from the drainage catheter placed in the subhepatic space, peritoneal signs, and elevations in liver function tests herald biliary tract complications. Sonography usually does not show biliary dilatation in the early postoperative period. Cholescintigraphy may not unmask subtle strictures, particularly in a marginally functioning liver. T-tube cholangiograms and endoscopic retrograde cholangiopancreatography (ERCP) are the gold standard if a choledochocholedochostomy has been performed. If a hepaticojejunostomy was employed for biliary reconstruction, a transhepatic cholangiogram may be necessary. Patency of the hepatic artery must be verified with ultrasound, since it is the only blood supply to the duct. Anastomotic strictures are sometimes amenable to dilatation with or without stenting. Complete disruptions, obstruction, and associated sepsis may warrant operative intervention and repeat anastomosis. *T-tube exit site leaks* may be managed with nasobiliary drainage or biliary stenting.

14.14. REJECTION

If technical and infectious factors have been ruled out, elevations of liver function tests in the early postoperative period are reflective of rejection. Percutaneous biopsy may be necessary to confirm the diagnosis. Usually treatment is with steroid boluses. Severe rejection may warrant OKT3 usage.

14.15. INTRA-ABDOMINAL BLEEDING

After liver transplantation, bleeding should not be a technical problem. On the operating table, all the anastomoses should be checked thoroughly and hemostasis should be complete. The coagulation status, as measured by PT, partial thromboplastin time (PTT), and thromboelastogram (TEG), should be acceptable, and all evidence of fibrinolysis or disseminated intravascular coagulation (DIC) corrected. Postoperatively, bleeding may ensue due to many possible causes. A clot may dislodge over a vessel, causing *hemoperitoneum*, but the most common cause is usually technical and hence avoidable with meticulous surgical technique, so this is relatively uncommon. If hemoperitoneum ensues, it is best to reexplore the patient and evaluate it, to avoid later problems of infected collections. In these cases of postoperative intra-abdominal hemorrhage, one must be very suspicious of primary allograft dysfunction. The patient may also develop *upper or lower gastrointestinal* (GI) *bleeding*, requiring endoscopic diagnosis and management and, rarely, laparotomy as, for instance, in bleeding from bowel anastomosis in cases reconstructed via Roux-en-Y choledochojejunostomy. Diagnosis of these conditions is based on the careful and continued monitoring of vital signs, hemodynamic status, serial hematocrit, and drain output. Prompt management, with replacement therapy and maintenance of hemodynamic stability while diagnostic endoscopy is performed or an operation is arranged, is essential for successful management of this condition.

Chapter 15

Postoperative Care in Kidney Transplantation

Radi Zaki and Shuin-Lin Yang

15.1. IMMUNOSUPPRESSION

The many regimens of immunosuppression vary mostly by center. The most common regimen at our Center is described here. Induction therapy with mono- or polyclonal antibodies (Daclizumab, Basiliximab, ATGAM®, Thymoglobulin®) varies from center to center. We commonly use Daclizumab induction, which has minimal side effects. The theory of induction prior to transplantation is a controversial topic. Induction therapy is not universally accepted and is dependent on center bias. It is generally accepted for high-risk patients, for patients with high panel reactive antibodies, prior transplants, and for African Americans. Maintenance immunosuppression consists of triple therapy, with a calcineurin inhibitor (cyclosporine or tacrolimus) plus mycophenolate or rapamycin, in addition to prednisone.

15.2. FLUID MANAGEMENT

Avoidance of prerenal azotemia in the perioperative period is of key importance in avoiding acute tubular necrosis (ATN). Fluid management is often aided by the use of central venous pressure or Swan–Ganz catheters. Since a large proportion of the patients have some cardiac disease, central venous pressure (CVP) monitoring is of key importance in aiding the use of fluids in high-output renal failure. Usual fluid replacement is milliliter-per-milliliter according to the cardiac filling pressures and is often adjusted to avoid pulmonary edema. Electro-lyte replacement is often needed in the form of potassium and magnesium in high-output renal failure. The use of preoperative antibiotics is indicated, as they are proven to decrease the rate of wound infections. The use of cephalosporin for 24–48 hours is sufficient.

15.3. HEMODIALYSIS

Hemodialysis should be avoided, if possible, due to volume contraction and subsequent hypotension, which can prolong delayed graft function by contribut-ing to ATN and potentially even cause graft thrombosis. The patient should have hemodialysis only if indicated, as in instances of severe hyperkalemia and/or respiratory compromise, with no evidence of resolving graft function.

15.4. HYPER- AND HYPOTENSION

Extreme variations in blood pressure should be avoided. Hypertension is more detrimental in the long-term survival of the graft, whereas hypotension is more of a threat in the immediate postoperative period and leads to ATN, vascular thrombosis of the graft, and delayed graft function. There is no clear consensus on the medical regimen for the treatment of hypertension in these patients. Calcium channel blockers (with the exception of nifedipine) cause elevation of cyclo-sporine (or tacrolimus) levels, complicating the postoperative picture. Acetyl-cholinesterase inhibitors may worsen renal function, giving rise to the suspicion of renal artery stenosis. Diuretics are often a good choice for treating these patients.

15.5. HYPERGLYCEMIA

Nutrition is usually started once bowel function has returned, commonly in the first postoperative day. A postoperative hyperglycemic state can be seen in three clinical scenarios. First, in those patients with preexisting diabetes mellitus (DM), hyperglycemia is exacerbated by steroids and can become quite labile and difficult to control. The demand for insulin is increased as renal function im-proves. These cases should always warrant consideration for pancreas transplanta-tion if the labile hyperglycemic state persists. The second type is a latent DM, which is unmasked by the high-dose steroids. This type tends to improve when the steroid dose is reduced and does not permanently require long-term insulin. DM is a major threat to the long-term survival of the renal allograft, thus stressing the development of new immunosuppressive regimens without steroids. Finally, tacrolimus and cyclosporine can also induce hyperglycemia, as they are toxic to the islet cells.

15.6. FOLEY CATHETER MANAGEMENT

The Foley catheter is left in place to monitor urine output and to allow the ureteroneocystostomy to heal and avoid urinary leaks. Patients that receive a Lich–Gregoir reimplantation (ureter anastomosed to a small hole in the bladder) may have the catheter removed on postoperative day 4 or 5. However, patients with ureteral reconstruction via the Ledbetter–Politano technique (bladder opened and ureter reimplantation inside the bladder), with atonic or very thin bladders, or with distal bladder obstruction, should have an indwelling Foley catheter for 7–10 days. Early removal of the Foley catheter decreases the incidence of urinary tract infections, which can be a devastating complication in an immunosuppressed patient. Patients are frequently placed on sulfa drugs postoperatively for a period of 4 months as prophylaxis for urinary tract infections.

15.7. VIRAL PROPHYLAXIS

Viral prophylaxis for cytometagalovirus (CMV) differs from center to center. High-risk patients, those that are CMV recipient negative/CMV donor positive, should be placed on intravenous gancyclovir and CMV hyperimmune globulin (Cytogam®), though the efficacy of Cytogam® in these patients has yet to receive support in the literature. Acyclovir is given to low-risk patients (i.e., CMV positive prior to transplant). Acyclovir also covers patients for herpes simplex types I and II.

15.8. SURGICAL COMPLICATIONS

Complications related specifically to the surgical procedure are common in these patients. Many of these complications are common to other surgical procedures, such as deep vein thrombosis, ileus, peptic ulceration, and so on. We discuss only those complications that are pertinent to the kidney transplantation procedure. Accordingly, hematomas and wound infections seen in the surgical site are relatively common, as patients frequently have uremic platelet dysfunction and are immunosuppressed. Careful hemostasis intraoperatively and adequate antibiotic prophylaxis should be employed to minimize this. Another type of collection is a lymphocele, which can displace the kidney and cause early or late allograft dysfunction. It is the result of leaking lymphatics at the operative site.

Meticulous surgical technique, with attention to tying off all perivascular lymphatics in the pelvis, is the best way to prevent this. Management of collections and infections requires drainage and appropriate antibiotics.

Acute tubular necrosis (ATN) manifests as lack of production of urine in the immediate postoperative period and has characteristic findings on allograft biopsy. Technically, all anastomoses are patent and the ureter is intact, but the graft has no urine production. Treatment is supportive and expected to continue for 2–3 weeks, and dialysis is frequently needed.

Technical issues include ureteric leaks and vascular problems. The latter are dealt with in detail later on. Ureteric leaks must be suspected early (within 2 weeks) and manifest as sudden pain (suprapubic or at the graft site), swelling, tenderness, urinary leakage from the incision, increase in serum creatinine, and decreased urine output. The most common site of ureteric leak is the anastomosis secondary to ischemia. Diagnosis by ultrasound reveals a perinephric collection that on sampling reveals a creatinine content greater than that of serum. Other diagnostic methods include computerized tomography (CT) and nuclear scans. Maneuvers to prevent this complication include minimization of the length of the ureter and proper procurement of the ureter to prevent vascular stripping. Technical errors, due to failure to construct a watertight anastomosis can also lead to possible ureteric leaks. Urinary leaks occur during brisk diuresis, either early on or in the first few weeks postoperatively. Treatment of this condition, which varies from center to center, may consist of percutaneous nephrostomy, a perinephric drain, and Foley catheter placement followed by an antegrade study for a possible stent placement. This is not a sound physiological approach for many reasons. First there is not significant hydronephrosis for a percutaneous nephrostomy. Second, there is an area of ureteric necrosis that will not respond to this treatment. Third, the ureter will heal with stricture formation. Finally, the placement of multiple drains and stents will increase the incidence of infectious complications in heavily immunocompromised patients. Urinary leaks, therefore, should always be managed surgically. A ureteric stent should be placed in the native ureter on the same side as the allograft in order to identify the native ureter if it is needed for reconstruction. This is due to the extensive amount of inflammatory reaction, which can make it difficult to find the native ureter. During the procedure, the ureter, as well as the bladder, should be debrided to healthy tissue. The reconstruction will depend on the clinical situation. If there is sufficient ureter length, a ureteroneocystostomy should be performed. If ureteric length is insufficient, an ureteropyelostomy or a cystopyelostomy with bladder advancement is an option. These should be created with the use of a double-J ureteric stent. The advantages of using the native ureters include avoiding vesicoureteral reflux.

Finally, other surgical complications can be seen, such as unilateral extremity edema and scrotal hydrocele. The former should prompt an investigation for deep vein thrombosis. In its absence, the condition is most likely due to the dissection and lymphatic division during the renal allograft implantation in the iliac fossa. The latter responds to drainage. Lymphoceles are discussed in Chapter 19.

15.9. COMPLICATIONS MANIFESTING IN ALLOGRAFT DYSFUNCTION

Allograft dysfunction in the early postoperative period presents as decreased urine output, with a failure of decrease in serum creatinine. In this setting, the following need immediate investigation: renal artery or vein thrombosis, ureteric leak, hematoma and bleeding, hyperacute rejection, and, finally, ATN. ATN causing delayed graft function will resolve with time, but the other conditions need immediate attention to salvage the allograft. With low urinary output, the central venous pressure (CVP) should be checked. With a low CVP, the patient should be fluid-challenged. If the CVP is high, a diuretic should be administered. If the patient fails to respond, a duplex ultrasound should be obtained. If intravascular flow is compromised or deficient, the patient should immediately return to the operating room for reexploration. If a collection is found, it should be aspirated and checked for fluid creatinine, definitive management of which is discussed below.

Hyperacute rejection or delayed hyperacute rejection is a condition in which preformed antibodies to human leukocyte antigens (HLA-Type I) result in vascular rejection. The onset of this phenomenon is usually immediate; however, it may not develop for a few days in delayed hyperacute rejection. The clinical manifestations are anuria, fever, abdominal pain, with tenderness over the graft, and swelling. Ultrasound shows an increase in the size of the allograft, with an increased resistive index. Renal scan shows minimal uptake of nuclear tracer. Biopsy shows glomerular endothelial injury and vascular thrombosis. The best treatment for this condition is prevention achieved by crossmatching the patient prior to transplant, which is standard practice of care. Otherwise, the only management of this condition is transplant nephrectomy.

Early rejection is a cellularly mediated event that may occur as early as the first week after transplantation. Patients commonly present with fever, decreased urinary output, elevated creatinine, occasional abdominal pain, and graft tenderness. This condition may be asymptomatic, with only an elevated creatinine. Ultrasound findings are consistent with increased size of kidney and an elevated ultrasound resistive index. Biopsy, indicated in these patients, shows diffuse lymphocyte infiltration in the interstitium, tubulitis, and glomerulopathy. The first line of therapy is high-dose steroids. If this fails, poly- or monoclonal antibodies should be used. The clinical significance of acute rejection is increased incidence of chronic rejection and subsequent earlier graft dysfunction and loss.

Toxicity of the calcineurin inhibitors (cyclosporine and tacrolimus) may also present with allograft dysfunction. Serum levels are usually elevated. Patients may have other signs and symptoms, such as hyperkalemia, hyperchloremic acidosis, and central nervous system (CNS) toxicity manifesting as tremors and seizures. Biopsy is characteristic, though not pathognomonic, and shows tubular vacuolization. Management is by decreasing the doses, provided that irreversible damage to the allograft has not occurred. The mechanism of nephrotoxicity is undetermined. The most plausible hypothesis is that the calcineurin inhibitor causes renal vasoconstriction.

15.10. VASCULAR COMPLICATIONS

Renal artery stenosis is a late complication most commonly associated with living related or living unrelated kidney transplants. The lower incidence in cadaveric transplants is related to the use of a Carrel patch. The Carrel patch is a cuff of aortic tissue surrounding the orifice of the renal artery in which one can sew the anastomosis to the patch, thus avoiding stenosis of the renal artery orifice. In general, the overall incidence is falling due to decreased use of the internal iliac artery as the inflow vessel for anastomosis to the allograft renal artery. Other surgical techniques that avoid this complication include the use of the external iliac artery as the site of anastomosis, or, as in living donors, arterial punch devices to create an end-to-side anastomosis. Symptoms of renal artery stenosis include hypertension or decreased allograft function. Ultrasound findings are consistent with increased peak systolic velocities. Patients given angiotensin-converting enzyme inhibitors will have aggravated blood pressure after administration of these agents. The gold standard for diagnosis of renal artery stenosis is a renal angiogram. Carbon dioxide angiography is an attractive alternative in this group of patients to avoid a dye load with potential nephrotoxicity.

Causes of renal artery stenosis include technical reasons (as mentioned earlier), rejection, atherosclerosis, and vascular clamp injuries. Treatment of this condition should include, as a first line of therapy, an attempt at percutaneous transluminal angioplasty, which has the best results. If this option fails, surgical reconstruction is indicated, though this procedure carries a significant rate of graft loss.

Renal artery and vein thromboses are relatively rare complications in the immediate postoperative period and are usually due to technical issues in vascular reconstruction. Patients usually have a dramatic clinical presentation of severe abdominal pain and tenderness over the allograft site, and worsening graft function. Doppler ultrasound findings will show no arterial flow consistent with arterial thrombosis. This presentation requires operative exploration. Renal vein thrombosis may present as late as the first week, with Doppler findings of increased arterial diastolic resistance, no venous flow, and increased allograft diameter. This condition is a surgical emergency.

Pseudoaneurysms in the kidney transplant recipient can be either anastomotic or intraparenchymal. Anastomotic pseudoaneurysms are frequently diagnosed by ultrasound and may present as fever or allograft dysfunction. Since they are frequently associated with infection, antibiotics are indicated. Surgical repair must be undertaken. Intraparenchymal pseudoaneurysms, usually secondary to a kidney biopsy, are best diagnosed by color flow Doppler scanning.

Arteriovenous fistulas occur mainly as a complication to percutaneous kidney biopsies. Most commonly, they are benign conditions that resolve spontaneously. Occasionally they cause persistent hematuria, hypertension, or allograft dysfunction. Diagnosis is confirmed with Doppler ultrasound, showing low diastolic resistance and visualization by color flow Doppler scanning. Treatment is indicated in the event of the aforementioned complications and consists of coil embolization of the isolated vessel. This is done with the risk of developing renal infarcts and worsening renal function, and should be performed by an experienced angiographer.

Chapter **16**

Postoperative Care in Pancreas Transplantation

Jorge A. Ortiz

The mortality for pancreas transplantation in the immediate postoperative period may be as high as 10–15%. For this reason, it is imperative that meticulous attention be paid to detail in both the operating room and the intensive care unit (ICU). Fortunately, recent advances in surgical technique and intensive care management have resulted in improved graft and patient survival.

16.1. GENERAL ICU CARE

The pancreas recipient leaves the operating theater in critical condition. The patient is intubated, with Swan–Ganz and arterial lines. Foley catheters and nasogastric tubes are used for bladder and gastric decompression. Most patients are extubated within 24 hours. The urinary catheter must remain for 7–14 days depending on the type of drainage for exocrine secretions and the type of ureteral implantation technique. The nasogastric tube remains until there is evidence of return of intestinal function. The patient is monitored in the early postoperative period for signs of ongoing hemorrhage, graft thrombosis, infection, leaks, pneumonia, and cardiovascular dysfunction. Serum amylase, lipase, and glucose are followed closely. Blood pressure, Swan–Ganz measurements, and blood gases are also monitored. It must be emphasized that the vast majority of Type 1 diabetics undergoing pancreas transplants have significant coronary disease (despite preoperative clearance), intestinal dysmotility, and increased susceptibility to infection.

16.2. IMMEDIATE COMPLICATIONS OF PANCREAS TRANSPLANTATION

Pancreas transplantation is a technically difficult procedure that has undergone significant evolution over the last decade. However, it is still associated with the highest surgical complication rate of all routinely transplanted solid organs. It shares complications with other major abdominal procedures (e.g., atelectasis, wound infection), as well as other transplant procedures (e.g., rejection, fungal and viral infections). However, it also exhibits a set of complications unique to this field. Surgical complications are responsible for 11–21% of all graft loss. Risk factors for surgical complications include advanced donor age and recipient obesity. Any or all of these complications may lead to graft loss and even death of the recipient.

16.2.1. Complications of Bladder Drainage

Fifty percent of transplant centers use duodenocystostomies for control of exocrine drainage. Proponents cite the ease of the anastomosis and the ability to follow urinary amylase to monitor for rejection as reasons to employ the bladder for drainage. However, a number of complications are unique to this technique.

16.2.1.1. Metabolic Acidosis and Dehydration

The loss of bicarbonate and water in the exocrine secretions of the pancreas into the bladder can lead to significant metabolic acidosis and dehydration. This dehydration can lead to dangerous hypotension, myocardial ischemia/infarction, and possible vascular thrombosis and graft loss. Due to the disordered metabolic milieu, life-threatening cardiac arrhythmias may also ensue. The treatment is vigorous hydration and mineral corticoids. Oral bicarbonate is also frequently necessary.

16.2.1.2. Hematuria

Blood in the urine is the most frequent urologic complication. It is usually self-limited. Proper hydration should be maintained. Management includes placement of a Foley catheter for bladder decompression and evacuation of blood clots. Dextran®, aspirin, and other inhibitors of proper clotting must be stopped. If bleeding persists, cystoscopic fulguration of bleeders may be necessary.

16.2.1.3.   Reflux Pancreatitis

This presents with elevated serum amylase and lipase. It is best treated with long-term urinary catheter placement and alpha-1 blockers. For recalcitrant cases, enteric conversion may be necessary.

16.2.1.4.   Duodenocystostomy Leak

The sudden onset of lower abdominal pain, fever, and leukocytosis, and elevations of amylase and creatinine, herald this complication. It may result from cytomegalovirus (CMV) infection, rejection or technical error. The diagnosis is confirmed with conventional cystogram, CT cystogram, or technetium scanning. For small leaks, expectant management is safest. For large disruptions or contined smaller leaks, reanastomosis or enteric conversion may be necessary.

16.2.1.5.   Other Urologic Complications

Other complications associated with bladder drainage include urinary tract infections, neurogenic bladder, urethral stricture, and balanitis. Persistence of these complications may warrant enteric conversion.

16.2.2.   Vascular Complications

16.2.2.1.   Arterial Graft Thrombosis

This presents in the first days to weeks after the procedure. It is the most common cause of nonimmunologic graft loss. The symptoms include a sharp rise in glucose and a drop in serum amylase levels. Amylase output in pancreatic juice or urine (if the bladder drained) disappears. The diagnosis is confirmed with Doppler ultrasound. The treatment is thrombectomy and revascularization. Some have tried interventional techniques of clot lysis. This may accompany rejection or infection. Risk factors include advanced donor age. Some centers use heparin, aspirin, or Dextran® as prophylaxis.

16.2.2.2.   Venous Graft Thrombosis

This presents within the first few weeks of the procedure. It manifests with a sharp rise in blood glucose and a rise in serum amylase levels. There is blood staining in the pancreatic juice or urine (if the bladder drained). The patient may also note pain and tenderness over the graft. This complication may result in graft loss. The treatment is venous thrombectomy, either operatively or with interventional radiologic techniques. Some centers will anticoagulate with heparin followed by coumadin and hope for recanalization of the vessel. Venous thrombosis may also accompany rejection or infection.

16.2.3. General Complications

16.2.3.1. Graft Pancreatitis

This may result from reflux or (more commonly in the immediate postoperative period) from ischemia reperfusion. Risk factors include donor premortem hypotension and rough handling during procurement. Graft pancreatitis presents with graft tenderness, high serum amylase and lipase levels, and maintained endocrine function. The treatment is supportive.

16.2.3.2. Intra-Abdominal Abscesses

These are seen more frequently with enteric drainage of exocrine secretions. They present 2–6 weeks postoperatively. Signs and symptoms include fever, leukocytosis, graft tenderness, and intact endocrine function. Treatment includes surgical and/or radiologic drainage with appropriate antibiotics.

16.2.3.3. Intrapancreatic Abscesses

These present 6–10 weeks postoperatively. Signs and symptoms include fever, graft tenderness, leukocytosis, and impaired endocrine function. Treatment is operative debridement and appropriate antibiotics. This frequently results in graft loss.

16.2.3.4. Pancreatocutaneous Fistula

Presentation is usually within 2 weeks of transplant. Auto digestion of the skin is seen, with a clear discharge high in amylase. The treatment is supportive.

16.2.3.5. Rejection

Rejection is responsible for 40% of graft failures. Exocrine function ceases before endocrine function. Therefore, there is a decrease in urinary amylase before endocrine dysfunction is noted. In simultaneous kidney–pancreas transplantation, a rise in serum creatinine signaling rejection of the kidney also signals pancreas rejection. Other methods of diagnosing pancreas rejection include pancreatic specific protein, interleukin 10, C-peptide, serum amylase–lipase levels, and magnetic resonance imaging. The gold standard for diagnosis is biopsy performed either percutaneously or via cystoscopy.

16.2.3.6. Hemorrhage

Continued intra-abdominal bleeding may necessitate reexploration. Hypotension, tachycardia, falling hematocrit, and a distended abdomen are all signs of continued bleeding that should be treated in the operating room. In a recent review, hemorrhage was the most common reason for reexploration in the tacrolimus era.

Chapter 17

Immunosuppression, Rejection Prophylaxis, and Other Pharmacotherapy of the Transplant Recipient

Cosme Manzarbeitia, Michael K. McGuire, and Rohit Moghe

17.1. INTRODUCTION

The goal of immunosuppression in transplant patients is to prevent acute and chronic rejection of the transplanted organ, while avoiding opportunistic infections and the adverse effects of immunosuppressive therapy (see Fig. 17.1). Combinations of immunosuppressants are used to affect different immune-system activators and to provide immunosuppressive synergy, using the lowest effective doses of immunosuppressants to reduce the potential for adverse drug events and drug interactions. Superiority of one regimen over another has not been demonstrated, and immunosuppressive protocols are largely program-specific. Familiarity with the immunosuppressants used in a particular programs' protocol is critical, along with a concordant understanding of therapeutic drug monitoring through serum levels and graft evaluation, adverse drug reaction monitoring, and judicious use of auxiliary medications that prevent and treat the consequences of immunosuppression. However, regimens should be flexible and take into account individual patient characteristics, such as the cause of liver failure, sensitization to histocompatibility antigens, side effects of the medications, exposure to previous

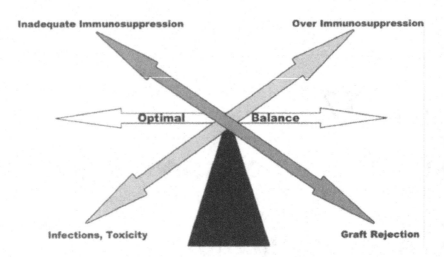

Figure 17.1. Balance of immunosuppression.

transplantation, and concomitant drug therapy. Medications used to prevent and treat the unwanted effects of immunosuppression should be chosen carefully, because these medications often interact with immunosuppressive agents. These interactions can often be exploited, however, by using lower doses of immunosuppressants. Some patients are more prone to the effects of immunosuppression than others; for instance, a recipient patient who lacks antibodies to cytomegalovirus (CMV) and receives an organ from a CMV-positive donor is more likely to develop symptomatic CMV than a recipient patient who has CMV antibodies. Finally, patient adherence and compliance to regimens are extremely important, and nonadherence is a common cause of organ rejection. Multidisciplinary transplant teams work collaboratively with patients to increase compliance with complicated medication regimens.

17.2. GLUCOCORTICOIDS

Corticosteroids reduce the capacity of antigen-presenting cells (APC-macrophages, B cells, etc.) to release interleukins 1 (IL-1) and 6 (IL-6), thus inhibiting lymphocyte proliferation and the release of IL-2, IL-3, IL-4, tumor necrosis factor (TNF), interferon alpha (INFα), and interferon gamma (INFγ). With the reduction in these cytokines, as well as the inflammatory eicosanoids and adhesion molecules on endothelial cells, the migration and phagocytosis capabilities of leukocytes, especially macrophages, are also inhibited. Lymphocytopenia, monopenia, and T-cell lysis also occur with glucocorticoids. The most commonly used corticosteroids in transplant protocols are methylprednisolone (Solu-Medrol®) given intravenously (IV) and prednisone (Deltasone® and others) given orally. Prednisone is absorbed after oral administration and converted hepatically to the active moiety, prednisolone. Methylprednisolone is about 1.25 times more potent than prednisone; it is often used for induction therapy intraoperatively and to treat episodes of acute rejection. In addition to concerns with long-standing corticosteroid therapy that suppresses the hypothalamic–pituitary–adrenal axis, slow discontinuation of therapy is desirable in order to manage cytokine rebound effect, because the receptors for cytokines are up-regulated in the presence of corticosteroids even though production is decreased. Although some programs dose steroids based on body weight, there is no convincing evidence that this is better than an empiric dosing strategy.

- *Dosage.*
  - Induction: 1000 mg IV day 1 (intraoperatively), tapering to 20 mg prednisone on day 6.
  - Maintenance: Usually 20 mg daily, tapering to 5 mg by the end of the first year, even discontinuing by 18-months posttransplant.
  - Acute rejection: 250–1000 mg IV on days 1, 2, and/or 3 tapering to 20 mg orally (PO) daily by day 6.
- *Important Side Effects.* Side effects include cushingoid effects such as fluid retention, hypertension, hyperglycemia, moon face, as well as bone demineralization and osteoporosis, gastritis, and/or peptic ulcers, cataracts, impaired wound healing, and increased susceptibility to infections.
- *Important Drug–Drug Interactions.* Interactions include increased metabolism in the presence of hepatic enzyme inducers (e.g., phenytoin, barbiturates, and rifampin) or decreased metabolism in the presence of hepatic enzyme inhibitors (e.g., grapefruit juice, cimetidine, macrolides, and "azole" antifungals [e.g., fluconazole]). Glucocorticoids may interfere with the effectiveness of vaccinations due to their inhibitory effect on leukocytes. Furthermore, steroids may reduce the ability of hypoglycemic agents to control blood glucose in diabetics.

17.3. CALCINEURIN INHIBITORS

17.3.1. Cyclosporine A (CyA)

The activation sequence of lymphocytes is altered by cyclosporin, which blocks humoral and cellular rejection mechanisms by binding to and forming a complex with immunophyllin protein and inhibiting the phosphatase activity of the enzyme calcineurin. This effect prevents the key steps in the G_0 and G_1 (gap) stages of cell cycle needed in initiating gene transcription necessary for the formation of lymphokines, especially IL-1 and IL-2. The result is inhibition of lymphocyte activation by T-helper cells and some loss of cytotoxic T-cell function, seemingly sparing T-suppressor mechanisms. Therapeutic drug levels are used to guide therapy. Target levels vary by organ and time after transplant. For example, in liver transplants, levels of 250–400 ng/mL (monoclonal TDX method) early on, with progressive decrease to maintenance levels of 150–250 ng/mL after 1 year are desirable. Lower levels are desirable for kidney transplants, due to the drug's nephrotoxicity. An important issue is the maintenance of adequate levels of the drug, due to the very variable (20–60%) bioavailability of CyA; best absorption is attained after a high-fat meal, although the microemulsified forms of CyA (Neoral®, Sangcya®, Gengraf®) are more readily bioavailable than the nonemulsified form (Sandimmune®). An IV formulation (Sandimmune®) is also available.

- *Dosage.*
  - ○ Induction: generally not used, may use low doses IV (1–2 mg/kg/24 h).
  - ○ Maintenance: 4–6 mg/kg/12 h PO.
- *Important Side Effects.* Side effects include nephrotoxicity, tremors, hirsutism, hypertension, gum hyperplasia, posttransplant lymphoproliferative disease (PTLD).
- *Important Drug Interactions.*
  - ○ Drugs that may potentiate nephrotoxicity (e.g., aminoglycosides, vancomycin).
  - ○ Drugs that may increase cyclosporine blood levels with potential for toxicity (drugs that inhibit the cytochrome P450 (e.g., "azole" antifungals, macrolides, 3-hydroxy-3-methylglutaryl coenzyme A (HMG-CoA) reductase inhibitors, grapefruit juice, diltiazem, verapamil). Sometimes these drugs are used in combination with cyclosporin to create "cyclosporin sparing regimens."
  - ○ Drugs that may decrease blood levels, leading to the potential for rejection (drugs that induce the cytochrome P450 (e.g., rifampin, antiepileptics, smoking, charcoal cooked foods)).

17.3.2. Tacrolimus (FK506, Prograf®)

The mechanism of action is similar to that of CyA but complexes with the intracellular protein, FKBP-12, leading to an inhibition of calcineurin; it is more potent than CyA. Therapeutic drug levels of 5–20 ng/mL during therapy are generally regarded as therapeutic in liver transplant patients. Tacrolimus is available in both PO and IV formulations; however, the IV formulation is very toxic and its use should be limited to patients not able to tolerate oral intake. It is not recommended to use CyA and tacrolimus simultaneously, as the risk of nephrotoxicity is compounded.

- *Dosage.*
  - ○ Maintenance: PO 0.15–0.3 mg/kg/q12h (every 12 hours).
  - ○ Acute rejection therapy (AR): Rarely used for this purpose. If so used, increase doses to achieve high trough levels (15–20 ng/mL).
- *Important Side Effects.* Toxicity is mostly neurologic, renal and endocrine (diabetogenic), similar to that seen with CyA.
- *Important Drug Interactions.* Since both drugs utilize the cytochrome P-450 enzyme system for metabolism, interactions are similar to those of CyA

17.4. ANTIMETABOLITES

17.4.1. Azathioprine (Imuran®)

A prodrug that is converted to 6-mercaptopurine, azathioprine produces nonspecific depression of DNA and RNA synthesis by inhibiting purine biosynthesis, in turn inhibiting T- and B-lymphocyte proliferation and differentiation. T lymphocytes are sensitive to inhibition of *de novo* purine synthesis because they lack efficient salvage pathways to maintain adequate intracellular levels. Azathioprine is frequently used in combination with other immunosuppressants, such as CyA and steroids.

- *Dosage.*
  - ○ Induction: Not used this way routinely; may be given at doses of 3–5 mg/kg as preoperative medication on call to operating room (OR).
  - ○ Maintenance: 1–2 mg/kg/d; adjust dose to white blood cell (WBC) level ≥ 4,000.
- *Important Side Effects.* Myelosuppression (leukopenia, thrombocytopenia, anemia), skin rash, nausea and vomiting, susceptibility to infections.
- *Important Drug Interactions.* Allopurinol, other myelosuppressive agents, angiotensin-converting enzyme (ACE) inhibitors.

17.4.2. Mycophenolate Mofetil (Cellcept®)

Mycophenolate is converted to an active form, mycophenolic acid, that blocks the *de novo* pathway for purine biosynthesis by inhibiting inosine monophosphate dehydrogenase (IMPDH), preventing conversion of inosine monophosphate (IMP) to guanosine monophosphate (GMP). This is especially important in T and B lymphocytes, therefore exerting a cytostatic effect in these cells. It is also used in conjunction with steroids and cyclosporine. Azathioprine and mycopheno-late mofetil are not to be taken simultaneously, as the risk of myelosuppression increases dramatically.

- *Dosage.* Maintenance: 500–1500 mg PO twice a day (bid), adjusted to WBC and side effects.
- *Important Side Effects.* Myelosuppression, diarrhea, infections, nausea, and gastric irritation.
- *Important Drug Interactions.* Acyclovir, gancyclovir and trimethoprim-sulfamethoxazole (Bactrim®; increased myelosuppression), antacids, and binding resins (e.g., cholestyramine, colestipol) cause decreased absorption.

17.5. ANTILYMPHOCYTE ANTIBODY PREPARATIONS

17.5.1. Muromonab-CD3 (Orthoclone OKT3)

A monoclonal antibody directed against the CD3 (T3) receptor present on the surface of T cells, muromonab-CD3 prevents antigen recognition. It also pro-motes lymphocyte lysis via complement fixation and/or antibody-dependent-cell mediated cytotoxicity. OKT3 is associated with the development of a severe cytokine release syndrome (CRS), resulting in a hyperdynamic state, with fever, tachycardia, and hypotension. This is due to the massive destruction of T cells with release of intracellular products. In the lungs, this produces an increased permeability and can lead to pulmonary edema in extreme instances. Management of this situation includes avoidance of fluid overload in the posttransplant patient, differentiation from septic states, and supportive therapy. It is important to con-sider that infection may coexist with this hyperdynamic state, and if it does not resolve within 48 hours, infection must be ruled out by usual means. In order to ameliorate this syndrome, premedication with methylprednisolone, diphenhydra-mine, and acetaminophen is indicated. Additionally, patients must have a clear chest X-ray for initiation of therapy, and hemodynamic monitoring is desirable.

The CD3 receptor appears when there is already some immunologic compe-tence. For this reason, it is frequently used for resistant rejection episodes, as T cells are the effector agents of acute allograft rejection. Since OKT3 is a murine antibody, antimurine antibodies limit the effectiveness of repeated courses. OKT3 is also a potent mitogenic factor for T cells, which explains the presence of recurrent rejection following its use, unless other drugs are used. Monitoring of its effectiveness includes CD3 counts at initiation and end of induction or rejection therapy. When treating rejection with antibody preparations, patients should be initially monitored in an ICU setting to avoid complications.

- *Dosage.*
  - ○ Induction: 5 mg IV every day (qd) for 7–10 days.
  - ○ AR therapy: 5 mg IV qd for 10–14 days.
- *Important Side Effects.* CRS, diarrhea, aseptic meningitis, encephalopathy, seizures, headaches, and infections.
- *Important Drug Interactions.* Doses of calcineurin inhibitors and other maintenance immunosuppressants should be reduced to avoid overimmunosuppression, potentially leading to increased risk of infections and/or malignancies.

17.5.2. Antithymocyte Globulins (ATGs)

ATGs are polyclonal antibodies (IgG) purified from the serum of animals immunized with human thymus lymphocytes that are directed against human lymphoid tissues. The two main preparations differ in their origin: Thymoglobulin® is derived from rabbit serum, and ATGAM® is derived from horse serum. The main risk associated with their use is anaphylaxis, as they are xenoantibodies. Their effectiveness varies between lots.

- *Dosage.*
  - ○ Induction: 15 mg/kg/d IV for 7–14 days (ATGAM®); 1.5 mg/kg/d IV for 7–14 days (Thymoglobulin®).
  - ○ AR therapy: 10 mg/kg/d IV for 10–14 days (ATGAM®); 1.5 mg/kg/d IV for 10–14 days (Thymoglobulin®).
- *Important Side Effects.* Anaphylaxis, serum sickness (usually seen 6–18 days after initiation of therapy), fever, chills, myelosuppression (leukopenia, thrombocytopenia), skin rash, nausea and vomiting, increased risk of infections.
- *Important Drug Interactions.* None known.

17.5.3. Interleukin 2 (IL-2) Receptor Antagonists

These are humanized monoclonal antibodies directed against the IL-2 receptor present at the lymphocyte surface. By inhibiting IL-2 binding, they inhibit the IL-2-mediated activation of lymphocytes. Because they are humanized chimeric antibodies, they do not elicit the CRS seen with the other antibody preparations. Two main compounds exist in this group: basiliximab (Simulect®) and daclizumab (Zenapax®), with similar safety and efficacy profiles. The difference is seen in the half-lives of the compounds, where the receptor saturation for basiliximab and dacluzimab is 36 and 120 days, respectively, at the recommended dosing. Currently the IL-2 receptor antagonists are only approved for use as induction agents in patients receiving renal transplant; however, they may be of benefit in other solid organ transplants.

- *Dosage.*
    - ○ Induction: Basiliximab → 20 mg IV given anywhere from preoperatively to within 2 hours of implantation, and repeated 4 days after transplantation; dacluzimab → 1 mg/kg given anywhere from preoperatively to within 24 hours of implantation, and repeated at 14-day intervals for four more doses.
- *Important Side Effects.* Potential for anaphylaxis, increased risk of infections.
- *Important Drug Interactions.* None reported.

17.6. SIROLIMUS (RAPAMUNE®)

Sirolimus has a structure similar to that of macrolide antibiotics and acts by forming a complex that binds the target of rapamycin [sirolimus] (TOR) protein, which in turn inactivates the proteins that bind tacrolimus (FKBP) and/or cyclosporine (cyclophyllin), therefore exerting a synergistic effect with these medications. It effectively prevents cytokine-driven T-cell proliferation, inhibiting progression from G_1 to S phases of the cell cycle. There is some evidence that sirolimus also inhibits antibody production. Even though serum levels (range: 8–12 ng/mL) can be obtained, these levels have not been correlated with either safety or efficacy.

- *Dosage.*
    - ○ Induction: 5-mg PO loading dose, followed by 2 mg PO qd afterwards.
    - ○ Maintenance: 2 mg PO qd.
- *Important Side Effects.* Thrombocytopenia, leukopenia, hyperlipidemia, increased susceptibility to infections.
- *Important Drug Interactions.* None reported to date, however, studies have shown that when cyclosporin is given concurrently with sirolimus, peak levels of cyclosporin are reduced. The manufacturer suggests separating doses with CyA by about 4 hours for best absorption, peak levels, and synergistic effects.

17.7. IMMUNOSUPPRESSIVE REGIMENS

Immunosuppressive medications can either be used alone or in combination for maintenance immunosuppression in any given patient; however, a multidrug approach is desirable for optimal immunosuppression. Using different immunosuppressive agents with different mechanisms of action and side effects has the advantage of enhancing immunosuppression and potentially minimizing adverse events associated with aggressive monotherapy. As Table 17.1 shows, some combinations or regimens are most likely to be useful in a given organ transplant model. Between transplant centers, there is great variability in dosing regimens, the type of transplant, as well as how well the donor organ HLA matches with the recipient. Most patients receive a triple-drug regimen for maintenance of immunosuppression, consisting of a calcineurin inhibitor, a steroid, and an antimetabolite; a fine line exists between under- and overimmunosuppression. In general, the level of immunosuppression is more likely to be aggressive in heart transplants, followed by lung, liver, pancreas, and kidney transplants. However, in renal and pancreatic transplants, cumulative rejection episodes can damage the graft and lead to chronic rejection. At the same time, these organs, especially the kidney, are more susceptible to the side effects (nephrotoxicity) of maintenance medications such a CyA and tacrolimus. Furthermore, rejection episodes are usually treated with higher doses of steroids and greater increases in baseline immunosuppression for organs such as liver or pancreas compared to kidney.

17.8.   OTHER MEDICATIONS

Patients who are maintained on immunosuppression for allograft survival are susceptible to many opportunistic diseases in addition to chronic diseases (e.g., hypertension, hyperlipidemia, etc.). Many drugs added to the preexisting regimen may interact with the immunosuppressants. Drug interactions should be managed by adjusting the doses of immunosuppressants to targeted levels. The following list of medications may be used in patients prior to or following transplant.

17.8.1.   Antivirals

Antiviral drugs are used to prevent and treat viral infections in immuno-compromised patients. Antivirals are used prophylactically at smaller doses or at larger doses for active treatment. For example, if the donor organ is positive for a virus (e.g., herpes simplex virus [HSV], CMV, and varicella–zoster virus [VZV]), and the patient is negative for that virus, antiviral medication(s) would be added to the regimen at full treatment doses to prevent the recipient from contracting the virus. Furthermore, if the donor organ is negative and the patient is positive for the virus, or if both the donor organ and the patient are positive, no viral prophylaxis or treatment would be needed (refer to institution-specific protocols).

- **Acyclovir (Zovirax®)**—Treatment of HSV and VZV (much less active against CMV): 200 mg PO bid for prophylaxis and up to 10 mg/kg PO three times a day (tid).

TABLE 17.1. Immunosuppression Regimens

| | Induction[b] | Maintenance[b] | Therapy of acute rejection | | | Therapy of chronic rejection |
			Severe	Moderate	Mild	
Liver transplant	1. OKT3 or antithymocyte globulins	1. CyA or Tacro (CNI), not both concurrently.	1. Steroid bolus followed by taper.	1. Steroid bolus followed by taper.	1. Increase baseline CNI and/or steroids; consider adding AZA, MMF, or Rapa.	1. Switch from CyA to Tacro.
	2. Steroid taper	2. Steroids (tapering schedule, even stopped after 1 year)	2. OKT3 or antithymocyte globulins	2. Increase baseline CNI, steroids; consider adding AZA, MMF, or Rapa.	2. Single or double (days 1 and 2) steroid boluses.	2. Add MMF or Rapa.
	3. IL-2 receptor blockers[a]	3. AZA or MMF (may be tapered or even stopped).	3. Increase baseline CNI, steroids; consider adding AZA, MMF, or RAPA.	3. OKT3 or antithymocyte globulins (rarely needed).		3. Retransplantation?
Comments:	Use either 1 or 3 along with 2.	Avoid quadruple ISX regimens to prevent infections or malignancies.	Use 1 first, followed by 2 if no response is seen, while simultaneously following with 3.	Use 1 while following with 2.	Frequently 1 suffices.	If 1 and 2 fail, retransplantation is a controversial approach for this group.

Kidney and pancreas transplant					
1. OKT3 or antithymocyte globulins or IL-2 receptor blockers.	1. CyA or Tacro	1. Steroid bolus followed by taper.	1. Steroid bolus followed by taper.	1. Steroid bolus followed by taper.	1. Switch from CyA to Tacro.
2. Steroid taper.	2. Steroids (tapering schedule to a low long-term maintenance dose).	2. OKT3 or antithymocyte globulins.	2. OKT3 or antithymocyte globulins.	2. Increase baseline CNI, steroids; consider adding AZA, MMF, or Rapa.	2. Add MMF or Rapa.
	3. AZA or MMF (may be tapered or even stopped).	3. Increase baseline CNI, steroids; consider adding AZA, MMF, or Rapa.	3. Increase baseline CNI, steroids; consider adding AZA, MMF, or Rapa.		3. Transplant nephrectomy and relisting.
	4. Rapa (used in combination wiht CyA or Tacro, may allow steroid dosage reduction or sparing).				
	Avoid quadruple ISX regimens to prevent infections or malignancies.	Acute rejection needs aggressive therapy to avoid graft damage and loss.	Acute rejection needs aggressive therapy to avoid graft damage and loss.	Acute rejection needs aggressive therapy to avoid graft damage and loss.	Nephrectomy reserved for graft-related complications, such as infections, etc.
Comments:	Use 1 and 2 simultaneously.				

Legend: CyA = cyclosporine A; AZA = azathioprine; MMF = mycophenolate mofetil; Steroids = glucocorticoids; Tacro = tacrolimus; Rapa = rapamycin; CNI = calcineurin inhibitors; ISX = immunosuppression.

[a] Still experimental.

[b] Many times, induction and initiation or maintenance therapy overlap.

- **Gancyclovir (Cytovene®)**—First-line agent for treatment of invasive CMV disease or CMV prophylaxis: 5 mg/kg IV q 12 h for 2–3 weeks, then 5 mk/kg IV qd for maintenance. Dose needs to be adjusted in renal failure and has dose-related myelosuppression.
- **Foscarnet (Foscavir®)**—Second-line for treatment of invasive CMV disease: 60 mg/kg IV q 8 h or 90 mg/kg q 12 h for 2–3 weeks; for treatment of acyclovir resistant VZV: 40 mg/kg q 8 h or 60 mg/kg q 12 h for up to 3 weeks. Dose should be adjusted in renal failure as it has additive nephrotoxicity.
- **Cidofovir (Vistide®)**—Third-line agent for invasive CMV disease: 5 mg/kg infused over 1 hour once weekly for two doses, then 5 mg/kg every 2 weeks. Due to potential for nephrotoxicity, hydrate the patient with 1 liter of normal saline solution 1 hour, and 2 g probenecid 3 hours prior to start of infusion.
- **CMV Hyperimmune Globulin (Cytogam®)**—Treatment provides passive immunity to CMV in transplant patients or CMV disease (reactivation of CMV). It is generally used in conjunction with antiviral agents (e.g., acyclovir, gancyclovir). In kidney transplant patients, an initial dose of 150 mg/kg is to be administered within 72 hours of the procedure, then an additional 100 mg/kg dose should be given every 2 weeks, for a total of five doses. In liver, lung, and heart transplant recipients, the initial dose is similar to that in kidney transplant recipients, then a dose of 150 mg/kg is given every 2 weeks (weeks 2–8) and a 100 mg/kg dose is given at weeks 12 and 16 after transplantation, for a total of seven doses. It is to be infused at a rate of 15 mg/kg/h for 30 minutes, and if that is tolerated, the rate can be increased to 30 mg/kg/h for the next 30 minutes, to a final infusion rate of 60 mg/kg/h.
- **Immunoglobulin (Gammagard®, Gamimune®, Sandoglobulin®)**—Treatment provides passive immunity against infectious disease when there are no vaccines available, and when patients have antibody deficiencies. Since all products are unique in their production, each product has its own dosing criteria. Gamimune is dosed at 100–200 mg/kg to a maximum of 400 mg/kg once monthly. Gammagard is dosed at 200–400 mg/kg once monthly, and Sandoglobulin is dosed at 200 mg/kg up to a maximum of 300 mg/kg once monthly.

17.8.2. Antibacterials

Patients on immunosuppressive regimens are at increased risk of developing bacterial infections, especially depending on the organ transplanted. Bacterial translocation with normal flora can cause clinically relevant bacterial infections. The most common cause of mortality following liver transplantation is infection.

- **Trimethoprim–sulfamethoxazole (Bactrim®, Septra®)** is used for prophylaxis of *Pneumocystis carinii* pneumonia (PCP), given as one double-strength (DS) tablet three times a week (Monday, Wednesday, Friday). Trimethoprim–sulfamethoxazole is also used to treat PCP. Alternatives for prophylaxis include pentamidine and dapsone.
- **Other: Macrolides, penicillins, cephalosporins, and quinolones** are not normally used for prophylaxis, but rather as treatments for presumed infections.

17.8.3. Antifungals

Patients on immunosuppression regimens are often at risk for developing fungal overgrowth, especially *Candida* sp. Patients may develop oral thrush, fungal esophagitis, or a vaginal yeast infection and need prophylaxis with antifungal medications; patients may also develop unusual fungal infections that do not normally occur in the general population.

- **Fluconazole (Diflucan®):** For treatment of *Candida* overgrowth, 100–200 mg PO daily. Prophylaxis: 100 mg daily to 100 mg weekly, depending on aggressiveness of immunosuppression.
- **Clotrimazole troche (Mycelex®):** For prophylaxis of *Candida* overgrowth, one 10 mg troche 4–5 times daily.
- **Nystatin (Mycostatin®):** For prophylaxis of fungal oral infections, 5 ml swish and spit, three to four times daily.
- **Amphotericin B (Fungizone®, Abelcet®, Ambisome®):** For the treatment of fungal infections caused by resistant *Candida* sp., cryptococcus, histomyces, blastomyces, and aspergillus. Due to the differences in amphotericin B preparations, the dosing will vary. The conventional amphotericin B (Fungizone®) is dosed at 0.5–1.0 mg/kg to a maximum of 1.5 mg/kg once daily infusion. The lipid formulations (Abelcet® and Ambisome®) of amphotericin B have less nephrotoxic effects, but there is no clinical difference between them. Abelcet® is dosed at 5 mg/kg once daily infusion, and Ambisome® is dosed at 1–5 mg/kg (depending on the sensitivity of the microorganism) once daily infusion.

17.8.4. Antihypertensives

Patients on immunosuppressive (especially CyA, tacrolimus, and glucocorticoids) regimens may develop hypertension that needs to be controlled with medications. Usually, calcium channel blockers (CCBs) are used, although there is place in therapy for angiotensin-converting enzyme (ACE) inhibitors. Nondihydropyridine CCBs diltiazem and verapamil interact with cyclosporin and tacrolimus, necessitating a lower dose of calcineurin inhibitor. However, verapamil may be nephroprotective when given before cyclosporin.

17.8.5. Hypoglycemic Agents

Patients on immunosuppression may already have previous history of diabetes mellitus, which may be worsened by some medications or may develop during maintenance therapy (e.g., glucocorticoids and/or tacrolimus). It may be necessary to initiate patients on hypoglycemic agents such as sulfonylureas, meglitinides, thiazolidinediones ("glitazones"), metformin, alpha-glucosidase inhibitors (e.g., acarbose or miglitol), or even insulin to maintain tighter control of blood glucose levels.

17.8.6. Lipid-Lowering Agents

A growing number of patients are starting to experience the effects of hyperlipidemia, especially since allograft survival has increased due to better immunosuppressive medications. In general, for patients who have plasma lipid abnormalities, agents such as HMG-CoA reductase inhibitors (for increased low-density [LDL] lipoprotein cholesterol), fibric acid derivatives (for increased triglycerides), bile acid-binding resins (for increased LDL and triglycerides), and niacin (for decreased high-density lipoprotein [HDL], and increased LDL and triglycerides) should be initiated to prevent the consequences of hyperlipidemia. For patients with mixed hyperlipidemia, a tailored program of blood lipid reduction may be necessary. Drug interactions with immunosuppressive regimens should be monitored closely.

17.8.7. Supplements

Patients may experience electrolyte abnormalities in addition to vitamin and nutritional deficits that may need to be supplemented.

Part V

Late Postoperative Complications and Outcomes

Chapter 18

General Late Complications in Transplantation

David J. Reich

Late postoperative complications following abdominal organ transplantation are related to side effects of chronic immunosuppression, disease recurrence, chronic rejection, and technical problems. As the outcomes after transplantation improve and recipients live longer, the late complications are seen more frequently. Long-term recipient survival depends on careful screening and management of the medical complications that these patients develop.

18.1. COMPLICATIONS OF IMMUNOSUPPRESSION

Long-term immunosuppressive therapy is a significant risk factor for renal dysfunction, hypertension, diabetes mellitus, hyperlipidemia, obesity, osteoporosis, malignancy, and infection. Although the toxicity profiles of individual immunosuppressive regimens differ, all transplant recipients are prone to develop these problems. As more immunosuppressant agents come into use, various combination regimens are being used to reduce toxicity.

18.1.1. Renal Dysfunction

The glomerular filtration rate falls continuously in recipients with long-term follow-up. Creatinine is typically elevated, between 1.5 and 2.5 mg/dL. Calcineurin inhibitors increased resistance in afferent glomerular arterioles and reduce renal blood flow. This process is exacerbated in the presence of concomitant diabetes or hypertension. Recurrent diseases may also aggravate renal dysfunction, such as recurrent glomerulosclerosis or glomerulonephritis in renal recipients, or glomerulonephritis and cryoglobulinemia in liver recipients with recurrent hepatitis C. Several medications compete with cyclosporine A and tacrolimus for cytochrome P450 metabolism, producing nephrotoxic levels of calcineurin inhibitors. Such medications include fluconazole, diltiazem, and verapamil. A common mistake is to administer erythromycin, often in combination with a nonsteroidal anti-inflammatory drug, to transplant recipients with upper respiratory tract infections; both drugs increase calcineurin inhibitor nephrotoxicity. Drugs that increase cytochrome P450 metabolism, such as many anticonvulsants, can cause nephrotoxicity if they are discontinued abruptly. Management of calcineurin inhibitor nephrotoxicity may include dose reduction and addition of nonnephrotoxic, newer immunosuppressive agents, including mycophenolate mofetil (CellCept; Roche, Nutley, NJ) and sirolimus (Rapamune; Wyeth-Ayerst, Wayne, PA).

Cyclosporine and tacrolimus are also notorious for causing renal tubular acidosis, associated with hypomagnesemia and hyperkalemia. Hypomagnesemia must be corrected, because it acts synergistically with cyclosporine and tacrolimus to lower the seizure threshold. Many transplant recipients require magnesium supplementation as well as a low potassium diet.

18.1.2. Hypertension

Although hypertension is common in transplant recipients, it is often easy to control with antihypertensive medications. Calcineurin inhibitors and steroids are the most significant causative agents among the immunosuppressant drugs, and cyclosporine causes hypertension more frequently than tacrolimus. These agents cause renal vasoconstriction resulting in increased reabsorption of sodium, fluid overload, and thus arterial hypertension. Management of post transplant hypertension requires diuretics and reduction of sodium intake if there is fluid overload. Furosemide is the agent of choice, because potassium-sparing diuretics exacerbate calcineurin-inhibitor-induced hyperkalemia. The preferred antihypertensives for use after transplantation are calcium channel blockers, which inhibit endothelin-induced vasoconstriction. It should be noted that diltiazem and verapamil, but not nifedipine, increase calcineurin inhibitor levels. Addition of a beta-blocker is often required. It has been shown that many transplant recipients tolerate complete steroid withdrawal, which decreases hypertension.

18.1.3. Diabetes Mellitus

Steroids increase gluconeogenesis and insulin resistance, and calcineurin inhibitors inhibit insulin release. Tacrolimus is more prone to cause hyperglycemia than is cyclosporine. Treatment of posttransplant diabetes mellitus requires dietary prudence, reduction of steroids, and/or calcineurin inhibitors and use of oral hypoglycemics or insulin.

18.1.4. Hyperlipidemia

Hyperlipidemia is commonplace in transplant recipients but tends to improve over time as immunosuppression is reduced. Posttransplant hyperlipidemia is of a mixed pattern, involving elevated cholesterol and/or triglyceride levels. Steroids and calcineurin inhibitors are causative. It has been shown that cyclosporine is a worse offender than tacrolimus. A major cause of mortality in long-term survivors after transplantation is cardiovascular-related disease; therefore, screening for, and managing, hyperlipidemia is important in this population. Therapy involves managing coexistent diabetes, hypertension, obesity, and smoking. Pharmacologic therapy may involve 3-hydroxy-3-methylglutaryl coenzyme A (HMG–CoA) reductase inhibitors, although these are rarely associated with myopathy and rhabdomyolysis, particularly in kidney recipients.

18.1.5. Obesity

Although many transplant recipients are malnourished before transplantation, excessive weight gain frequently occurs after transplantation. Risk factors include increased caloric intake, decreased physical activity, corticosteroid use, and coexistence of diabetes mellitus. Managing obesity is particularly important because this complication is itself a significant risk factor for development of the other complications of hypertension, diabetes mellitus, hyperlipidemia, and osteoporosis. Managing posttransplant obesity requires dietary restriction, exercise, and steroid reduction. Although there is interest in the use of medication to treat obesity, further studies are required to evaluate the safety of such therapy in this patient population.

18.1.6. Osteoporosis

The most common presentation of posttransplant osteoporosis is an atraumatic fracture of trabecular bones, such as vertebrae and ribs. Avascular necrosis commonly affects the femoral heads or the knees. Immunosuppressive therapy is a risk factor for postoperative loss of bone mass. Corticosteroids cause increased bone reabsorption, decreased bone formation, and calcium malabsorption. Calcineurin inhibitors also cause high bone turnover. The most frequently used tool for determining the presence of significant osteoporosis is dual energy X-ray absorptiometry (DEXA) scanning. Magnetic resonance imaging (MRI) is the test of choice for determining the presence of avascular necrosis. Management options include weight loss, exercise, and pharmacotherapy, including vitamin D and calcium supplementation, and hormone therapy or use of biphosphonates. Osteonecrosis may require prosthetic hip or knee replacement, which can be performed safely in transplant recipients.

18.1.7. Posttransplant Malignancies

Immunosuppressive medications do not increase the frequency of most common malignancies but do significantly increase the risk of lymphoma, skin cancer, and some rare malignancies, including Kaposi's sarcoma and carcinoma of the cervix, external genitalia, and perineum.

18.1.7.1. *Posttransplant Lymphoproliferative Disease*

PTLD is related to infection with Epstein–Barr virus. Most PTLD arises from B lymphocytes. Patients at highest risk for developing PTLD are children, recipients who were seronegative for Epstein–Barr virus and received organs from donors that were seropositive, and patients who required the use of monoclonal antibody immunosuppressive therapy (OKT3). PTLD, in contrast to nontransplant-related lymphomas, is often extranodal, presenting in such places as the gastrointestinal tract, lung, or central nervous system. Therapy involves decreasing immunosuppressive medications, and use of antivirals and sometimes chemotherapy or radiotherapy.

18.1.7.2. *Skin Cancer and Kaposi's Sarcoma*

Skin cancer, including squamous cell carcinoma, melanoma, and basal cell carcinoma, occurs up to 20 times more frequently in transplant recipients than in the general population. In general, skin cancer is more aggressive in transplant recipients than in the general population. Transplant recipients should avoid sun exposure and undergo routine skin evaluations. Kaposi's sarcoma may present with bluish skin lesions or may affect the oropharynx, lung, or other viscera. Treatment involves decreasing immunosuppression and may also involve chemotherapy or radiotherapy.

18.1.8. Posttransplant Infections

Patients with long-term follow-up after organ transplantation are only at slightly increased risk for developing common bacterial or viral infections. However, they are at increased risk for opportunistic infections. The usual viral culprits are DNA herpes viruses, most importantly cytomegalovirus, and also Epstein–Barr virus, herpes simplex virus, and varicella. Cytomegalovirus may present with fever, malaise, leukopenia, hepatitis, esophagitis, enterocolitis, pneumonitis, or retinitis. Treatment involves immunosuppression reduction and gancyclovir, which is highly therapeutic. The most common fungal infections in transplant recipients include candida, aspergillus, cryptococcus, and histoplasmosis. Risk factors for these opportunistic infections include heavy immunosuppressive regimens, often in the face of allograft dysfunction, and use of broad-spectrum antibiotics. Aspergillosis most often presents with respiratory symptoms, and cryptococcus, most often with meningitis. These fungal infections are treated with fluconazole or amphotericin B, but mortality rates are high. Other opportunistic infections include *Pneumocystis carinii*, mycobacterium, and the bacteria *Legionella*, *Nocardia*, and *Listeria*. Patients with long-term follow-up who still require heavy immunosuppression should be maintained on chronic antifungal as well as antiviral prophylaxis, with agents such as oral mycelex, vaginal nystatin and acyclovir. Trimethoprim–sulfamethoxazole is used for *Pneumocystis carinii* pneumonia prophylaxis.

Transplant recipients should receive annual pneumococcal and influenza vaccines. The use of live attenuated viral vaccines is contraindicated in the face of high-level immunosuppression.

18.2. DISEASE RECURRENCE, CHRONIC REJECTION, AND TECHNICAL PROBLEMS

18.2.1. Disease Recurrence

Transplant recipients may be susceptible to recurrence of their original disease. Some recurrent diseases are mild, whereas others have a propensity to cause allograft failure. Liver transplant recipients may develop recurrence of hepatitis C, hepatitis B, hepatocellular carcinoma, alcoholic liver disease, or one of the autoimmune hepatitides (see Chapter 19). Kidney recipients may develop recurrence of diabetic nephropathy, focal segmental glomerulosclerosis, membranoproliferative glomerulonephritis, immunoglobin A (IgA) nephropathy, hemolytic uremic syndrome, or systemic lupus erythematosus (see Chapters 19 and 21).

18.2.2. Chronic Rejection

Chronic rejection involves progressive deterioration of allograft function. The process is based on immune humoral reactivity leading to tissue fibrosis; it may be exacerbated by nonimmunologic factors such as ischemia reperfusion injury, cytomegalovirus infection, and immunosuppression induced hyperlipidemia, diabetes, and hypertension. Heavy immunosuppression with tacrolimus, mycophenolate mofetil, and/or sirolimus may reverse chronic rejection in the early phases. Renal recipients are particularly prone to chronic rejection. They suffer decreased glomerulofiltration rates, proteinuria, and uremia. Histopathology reveals vascular intimal thickening and obliteration, glomerulosclerosis, tubular atrophy, and interstitial fibrosis. Liver recipients can also develop chronic rejection. They develop hepatic arteriolar thickening, loss of bile ductules and hepatic fibrosis, resulting in jaundice, loss of synthetic function, and portal hypertension (see Chapter 19 for a detailed discussion about chronic rejection in kidney and liver transplantation).

18.2.3. Technical Problems

Discussion of the technical problems that occur posttransplantation is found in Chapter 19.

Organ-Specific Late Complications in Transplantation

David J. Reich, Cosme Manzarbeitia, Radi Zaki,
Jorge A. Ortiz, and Sergio Alvarez

19.1. LIVER TRANSPLANTATION

Late complications specific to liver transplantation include technical complications, recurrent liver disease, and chronic hepatic rejection, in addition to the side effects of long-term immunosuppression that affect recipients of any type of organ transplant (discussed in Chapter 18). Evaluation of allograft dysfunction in the liver recipient with long-term follow-up requires screening for hepatic artery thrombosis or stenosis, biliary problems, recurrent disease, rejection, and infection. All of these problems may present with similar findings and laboratory abnormalities. Initial workup routinely includes duplex ultrasound, cholangiogram, liver biopsy, pan cultures, and serology testing.

19.1.1. Technical Complications

Technical complications that present late posttransplant involve the biliary and hepatic vascular trees.

19.1.1.1. Biliary Complications

After the early posttransplant period, biliary complications involve bile leaks, usually from the T-tube tract, and anastomotic stenosis of the choledocho-choledochostomy or choledochojejunostomy.

19.1.1.1a. Biliary Leak.   Spontaneous bile leaks from the anastomosis or elsewhere are unusual late posttransplant because of the scarring process. However, patients may suffer a bile leak from the T-tube exit site, approximately 3 months posttransplant. Most centers that use T tubes to stent the biliary anastomosis bring the long limb of the tube out through the recipient bile duct. This is removed approximately 3 months posttransplant, following a normal cholangiogram. T tubes used in the nontransplant setting are generally removed long before 3 months. However, transplant recipients do not form a mature tract until several months posttransplant because of heavy immunosuppression. Occasionally, 3 months is still not long enough to form a mature tract, and after T-tube removal, bile that leaks into the abdominal cavity causes peritonitis. Most leaks are self-limited and the only therapy required is hydration and antibiotics. Sometimes, severe peritonitis and even septic shock develop, necessitating emergent endoscopic retrograde cholangiopancreatography (ERCP) and nasobiliary or internal stenting. Surgery for a T-tube tract leak is only rarely required. This complication is one of the reasons that more and more programs perform the choledochocholedochostomy without T-tube stenting.

19.1.1.1b. Biliary Stricture.   The majority of biliary complications that present late posttransplant are related to biliary ischemia from hepatic artery stenosis or thrombosis, or from low flow state related to sepsis. The biliary tree receives blood supply predominantly from the arterial rather than the portal vascular system. The donor duct receives arterial supply via the hepatic artery. In the nontransplant setting, the duct is also supplied by the paraduodenal arcades, but in transplant recipients these arcades are severed during the hepatectomy. Therefore, the allograft distal bile duct is particularly prone to ischemia. Biliary ischemia in the patient with long-term follow-up usually presents aas a stricture of the duct-to-duct or biliary–enteric anastomosis. Patients develop insidious allograft dysfunction or overt jaundice and/or cholangitis. ERCP (in the case of a duct-to-duct anastomosis) or percutaneous transhepatic cholangiography (PTC) (in the case of a biliary–enteric anastomosis) is diagnostic and may allow for stenting and balloon dilatation of the stricture. Failure of balloon stricturoplasty necessitates surgical revision, namely, conversion of a duct-to-duct anastomosis to a Roux-en-Y choledochojejunostomy or revision of a choledochojejunostomy. Sometimes, biliary ischemia affects the more proximal biliary tree. In the most extreme situation, patients develop secondary sclerosing cholangitis, which, if progressive, is an indication for retransplantation. An important point to remember is that a patient who presents with biliary problems posttransplantation requires evaluation of not only the biliary tree but also the hepatic artery.

19.1.1.2. Vascular Complications

Vascular complications that affect liver recipients with long-term follow-up include thrombosis or stenosis of the hepatic artery or portal vein.

19.1.1.2a. Hepatic Artery Thrombosis and Stenosis. Approximately 4% of transplant recipients develop hepatic artery thrombosis, and half the time this occurs in patients with long-term follow-up. Risk factors for hepatic artery thrombosis include pediatric cases (because of small vessel size), vascular reconstructions (such as for a donor accessory right hepatic artery originating from the superior mesenteric artery), anastomotic technical imperfections, intimal injuries (such as from clamping, traction, or long cold ischemia), poor inflow, and high outflow resistance (such as during rejection or other forms of allograft dysfunction). Recently, more attention is being paid to the role of hypercoagulable states predisposing to hepatic artery thrombosis. Hepatic artery thrombosis presents with a spectrum of manifestations ranging from insidious allograft dysfunction to overt hepatic necrosis with fulminant liver failure. The most common presentation involves biliary complications, including Gram-negative sepsis, anastomotic stricture, or intrahepatic bile lakes. Unlike hepatic artery thrombosis in the early posttransplant period, which is often diagnosed shortly after onset and is therefore amenable to repair, late hepatic artery thrombosis is usually diagnosed after a delay and is not amenable to repair; even if revascularization is possible, it is not safe to reperfuse chronically necrotic tissue. Some recipients tolerate hepatic artery thrombosis, whereas others require biliary interventions (such as stricturoplasties or biloma drainages), and approximately half require retransplantation. Many programs perform periodic surveillance ultrasonography, even long-term, after transplantation, to screen for hepatic artery stenosis. Hepatic artery stenosis is amenable to angioplasty, or surgical revision, prior to development of full-blown hepatic artery thrombosis.

19.1.1.2b. Portal Vein Thrombosis and Stenosis. Portal vein thrombosis and stenosis are rare, occurring in less than 1% of liver transplant recipients. Acute thrombosis may cause fulminant liver failure. In other cases, patients present insidiously with manifestations of portal hypertension, including ascites or variceal hemorrhage. Acute thrombosis may be amenable to emergent thrombectomy. The cases that present insidiously often require portosystemic shunting, either surgically or with transjugular intrahepatic portosystemic shunt (TIPS). Risk factors for portal vein thrombosis include pretransplant portal vein thrombosis, hypercoagulable states, low flow states, and recurrent hepatic fibrosis or cirrhosis.

19.1.2. Chronic Hepatic Rejection

The hallmark of chronic rejection in liver recipients is biliary ductular necrosis, termed "ductopenia" and "vanishing bile duct syndrome," which results in progressive jaundice. The ducts suffer direct lymphocytotoxic injury as well as ischemia from the obliterative vasculopathy caused by antibody-mediated intimal damage of hepatic arterioles. In the late phase of chronic rejection there is diffuse hepatic fibrosis. Allograft function deteriorates, marked by cholestasis and ultimately, loss of synthetic function and portal hypertension. Putative risk factors include human leukocyte antigen (HLA) mismatching and nonimmunologic factors such as ischemia reperfusion injury and cytomegalovirus infection. Heavy immunosuppression with tacrolimus, mycophenolate mofetil, and/or sirolimus may reverse chronic rejection in the early phases. Advanced chronic rejection is an indication for retransplantation.

19.1.3. Recurrent Disease after Liver Transplantation

Many diseases may recur after liver transplantation; in some cases, these may recur after liver transplantation; in others, there may be no immediate impact on patient or graft function, at least in the short term.

19.1.3.1. Metabolic Liver Disease

When the metabolic abnormality is primarily within the liver, transplantation will be curative for metabolic disease; transplantation, at present, is indicated only where there is also significant liver disease (e.g., hemophilia with end-stage hepatitic C virus [HCV] infection). Such indications include alpha1-antitrypsin deficiency, antithrombin-III deficiency, protein C deficiency, protein S deficiency, Wilson's disease, tyrosinosis, Byler's disease, galactosemia, hemophilia A and B, and Crigler–Najjar syndrome. Where the disease process is extrahepatic, liver replacement is not always indicated. However, when the disease recurs, transplantation is sometimes indicated, as the effects of disease can be modified, as with genetic hemochromatosis and congenital erythropoietic porphyria. In patients grafted for cystic fibrosis, the disease may affect the graft but medium-term survival is good. In conditions such as the sea-blue histiocyte syndrome or Gaucher's disease, liver replacement is not indicated.

19.1.3.2. Autoimmune Liver Disease

Most autoimmune liver diseases will recur in the allograft but have little impact in the short and medium term. *Primary biliary cirrhosis* recurs in the allograft in 20% of patients at 5 years and 45% at 51 years. Some have found that recurrence is greater in those on tacrolimus compared with cyclosporine. The role of ursodeoxycholic acid (UDCA) in this situation is unclear. *Autoimmune hepatitis*, which may recur, especially if corticosteroids are withdrawn, usually responds rapidly to reintroduction of steroids, with no adverse, long-term impact. In *primary sclerosing cholangitis* (PSC), diagnosing recurrence is difficult since differentiation between recurrent primary disease and *de novo* secondary disease may be difficult. PSC recurs in about 45% of patients at 5 years and may lead to cirrhosis, requiring retransplantation.

19.1.3.3. Viral Hepatitis

The *hepatitis A virus* may reinfect the graft, but in the few cases reported, there have been no significant consequences. As for the *hepatitis B virus* (HBV), until recently, recurrent HBV meant that those who were HBV DNA positive prior to transplantation were contraindicated for transplantation. Those who were DNA negative were treated with hepatitis B immune globulin (HBIg). Now, patients are treated with lamivudine for 6 weeks prior to transplantation, until HBV is reduced to less than 1 million copies/ml or undetectable. Follow-up after transplantation is with both lamivudine and HBIg; the optimal dose and duration of HBIg treatment is uncertain, but some centers aim to maintain levels above 100 units/ml forever or offer vaccination. Development of resistant mutants is an increasing problem. The role of other antiviral therapies, such as gancyclovir, adefovir, or famciclovir, is uncertain at this time. The *hepatitis C virus* (HCV) almost invariably recurs after transplantation but the extent of the graft damage is variable. Survival in the short term is not significantly affected, but there are concerns regarding long-term recurrence, as cirrhosis at 5 years occurs in 8–25% of patients. Several factors have been variably implicated in recurrence, including genotype (1b), viral load, HLA match, degree of immunosuppression, quasi-species, and recipient age. Patients grafted more recently for HCV appear to develop graft fibrosis more quickly; the reasons for this are uncertain. The roles of interferon and/or ribavirin are uncertain: Concerns about inducing chronic rejection need to be balanced against any therapeutic benefit. Until recently, *HIV and AIDS* were contraindications for transplantation; the advent of successful control of viral replication has led some centers to transplant HIV patients. Outcomes are variable.

19.1.3.4. Other Indications

A return to alcohol will lead to recurrent *alcoholic liver disease* in a small proportion of cases, although, overall, 1- and 5-year survival is no different in this cohort of patients. Pretransplant abstinence, often necessary to determine if the liver will recover enough to avoid the need for transplantation, is a relatively poor indicator for future abstinence. *Nonalcoholic steatohepatitis* (NASH) is occasionally an indication for transplantation. Recurrence of NASH has been identified after transplantation and may be associated with progressive fibrosis in the graft. This is more common when the underlying cause of the NASH (such as obesity or jejunal–ileal bypass) has not been altered. *Budd–Chiari syndrome*, once a major indication for transplantation, is less common now, due to the introduction of other treatments. There is a 30–40% probability of further thrombosis despite the use of anticoagulation. The presence of an underlying disorder will affect the need for transplantation. Post liver transplantation *cancer* is usually persistence rather than recurrence. For liver cell cancer (HCC), hepatocellular carcinoma, the probability of recurrence is predicted by the size and number of nodules (most imaging modalities underestimate both), the presence of capsular penetration, lymph node involvement, and vascular invasion. Options to treat the cancer prior to or during surgery have had little impact. Cholangiocarcinomas are very difficult to detect prior to transplantation and are rarely cured, although aggressive approaches with chemo- and brachytherapy have been associated with a good outcome in selected patients at the Mayo Clinic. The only secondary cancers that may be indications for liver transplantation are the symptomatic endocrine tumors in which worthwhile palliation can be achieved.

19.2. KIDNEY TRANSPLANTATION

Most technical complications in the kidney transplant recipient occur during the early postoperative period (i.e., within the first month after transplant). A few of these, however, may be seen later on in the course of treatment and are briefly described here. By and large, the major cause of morbidity and kidney graft loss in the late postoperative period is the development of chronic, irreversible rejection. Finally, many of the long-term complications of immunosuppression have already been described in Chapter 18 and are not repeated here.

19.2.1. Surgical Complications

19.2.1.1. Lymphocele

Lymphoceles are collections of lymphatic fluid in the preperitoneal and retroperitoneal space, and their incidence ranges from 10% to 15%. They are caused by disruption of the lymphatics lying along the course of the iliac vessels during preparation for implantation of the allograft in the retroperitoneal space; this complication is not seen with intra-abdominal placement of the allograft. Prevention centers on meticulous ligation of the lymphatics around the iliac vessels versus sharp dissection around the lymphatics. Lymphoceles may cause allograft dysfunction by creating venous obstruction, ureteric obstruction, infection, and lower extremity pain and swelling. The clinical presentation is of swelling and tenderness over the graft, lower extremity swelling, a rise in serum creatinine and a decrease in urine output, and are usually seen within the first 3 to 6 months after transplantation. Diagnosis can be made by ultrasound revealing a perinephric collection. The collection should be sampled for creatinine and protein content. Compared to serum, the fluid has a higher protein content and an equal creatinine. Treatment is indicated in large, symptomatic, or complicated lymphoceles. No surgical treatment is indicated for small asymptomatic lymphoceles. The first line of therapy is percutaneous drainage with a closed suction system. Once the drainage decreases, the drain may be removed. If the drainage does not decrease, sclerosing agents in the form of alcohol or betadine can be used. If the lymphocele recurs, surgical management is indicated. Surgical management consists of internal drainage, which can be performed by an open technique in which the lymphocele is drained into the peritoneal cavity and omentum is placed in the lymphocele cavity. This can also be achieved laparoscopically to create a peritoneal window.

19.2.1.2. Ureteric Stenosis

The ureteric anastomosis is the Achilles' heel of kidney transplantation. There is a high risk of ischemic injury, a result of the segmental blood supply to the ureters. Vascular disruption of the ureters is dependent on the technique of the harvesting surgeon to maintain a significant amount of tissue around the ureters during extraction. Ureters are more vulnerable to ischemic injury during living related or living unrelated versus cadaveric extractions. Ureteric leaks have been discussed previously. Ureteric stenosis may be a manifestation of ischemia or rejection, or secondary to extrinsic obstruction. Examples of extrinsic obstruction are lymphocele or ureteric kinking. Common clinical presentations may be asymptomatic allograft dysfunction presenting with proteinuria, increasing creatinine, and proteinuria. The cause of this dysfunction will be identified on ultrasound as hydronephrosis. The diagnostic gold standard is an antegrade nephrogram via percutaneous nephrostomy or a retrograde pyelogram. Retrograde pyelograms can be extremely difficult to complete due to an obscure ureteric orifice as a result of implantation. Therapeutically, the stricture can be dilated and a double-J stent can be passed. The stent can subsequently be removed in 2 weeks to a month. This is very effective treatment for strictures less than 2 cm in length. For strictures greater than 2 cm in length, surgical intervention is required. For strictures due to extrinsic obstruction, the cause should be treated.

19.2.1.3. Renal Artery Stenosis

This is the most common late vascular complication, most often associated with living related or living unrelated kidney transplants, and has been described in detail in Chapter 15.

19.2.2. Chronic Rejection

Chronic rejection is the major cause of graft loss in renal transplantation. The term "chronic rejection" is a misnomer; the proper term should be "chronic allograft nephropathy." Histological findings of chronic rejection are interstitial fibrosis, tubular atrophy, glomerular proliferation, and sclerosis, as well as arterial intimal thickening (see Chapter 21). The etiology is multifactorial. Immunologic factors contributing to chronic rejection are repeated episodes of acute rejection, which occur several months after transplantation, inadequate immunosuppression (iatrogenic or due to noncompliance), and HLA mismatching. The nonimmunologic factors are hypertension, delayed graft function, cold ischemic time, donor age > 55 years, and hyperlipidemia. Chronic allograft nephropathy is neither prevented nor treated with current, available immunologic medications. An important factor for managing a patient with chronic allograft nephropathy is to rule out other causes of allograft dysfunction, including acute rejection, calcineurin inhibitor toxicity, and recurrence of preexisting diseases. Chronic allograft nephropathy presents as a slow, insidious process of deteriorating creatinine clearance, proteinuria, and hypertension. However, the secondary causes of allograft dysfunction usually have an acute onset, presenting with more rapid allograft deterioration.

19.2.3. Disease Recurrence

Recurrence of the primary kidney disease is rare, accounting for only 1% of cases of late allograft dysfunction. In general, kidney recipients may develop recurrence of diabetic nephropathy, focal segmental glomerulosclerosis, membranoproliferative glomerulonephritis, immunoglobin A (IgA) nephropathy, hemolytic uremic syndrome, or systemic lupus erythematosus (see Chapter 21).

19.3. PANCREAS TRANSPLANTATION

19.3.1. Rejection

Acute rejection in simultaneous kidney–pancreas (SPK) transplantation is usually diagnosed by a rapid increase in serum creatinine, along with a decrease in urinary amylase (25% from the baseline) fall in urinary pH, and, finally, a rise in plasma glucose. Exocrine function is impaired well before endocrine manifestations are noted. Other monitoring tests include magnetic resonance angiography, pancreas-specific protein, and interleukin-10. However, the gold standard for the diagnosis of rejection is biopsy, though it is not commonly performed.

The incidence of acute pancreas rejection episodes is significantly lower in SPK compared with pancreas after kidney (PAK) transplant and pancreas transplant alone (PTA). Nowadays the incidence of rejection has decreased secondary to the use of new immunosuppressive drugs (tacrolimus, mycophenolate, anti-IL-2 antibodies, etc.). Graft failure rates secondary to immunologic reasons for SPK at 1, 2, and 3 years are 2%, 3%, and 5%, respectively; for PAK, 9%, 14%, and 20%, respectively; and for PTA, 16%, 18%, and 30%, respectively.

Chronic rejection is characterized by a progressive increase of blood glucose levels or increased insulin requirements, with a continued decline in urinary amylase and C-peptide concentration in patients with multiple previous acute rejection episodes. Data from the University of Wisconsin (*Ann Surg* 1998;*228*, 3) demonstrate that minimizing HLA mismatches improves the long-term survival in SPK recipients by decreasing the incidence of chronic rejection.

19.3.2. Urologic Complications

The most frequent late complications in kidney–pancreas transplantation are urologic in nature. These are usually seen in pancreata drained into the bladder, and management of complications frequently involves conversion to enteric drainage. The conversion rate for severe urologic complications ranges between 15% and 20%.

19.3.2.1. Hematuria

Early hematuria is due to suture line bleeding and has an incidence rate of 17%. Chronic hematuria is usually the result of ulcerations in the duodenal segment or from bladder stone formation in the suture or staple line. It can also be related to the granulation tissue observed in the area of the anastomosis. It requires intervention in approximately 30% of cases. Treatment is with Foley catheter placement, irrigation, and/or cystoscopy for evacuation of clots and fulguration of bleeders.

19.3.2.2. Duodenal–Bladder Leaks

Commonly observed in the first 6 months posttransplant, duodenal–bladder leaks can be seen in up to 15% of cases and can result from technical anastomotic breakdown, acute or chronic rejection, and cytomegalovirus (CMV) infection.

19.3.2.3. Urethral Strictures

This complication usually results from urethritis and is seen in 2.8% of cases. It is usually observed months to years postsurgery. Enteric conversion is necessary if short-term therapy with Foley catheterization fails.

19.3.2.4. Chronic Urinary Tract Infections (UTIs)

This is the most frequent complication (62.5%) of patients induced by the irritant effect of exocrine secretions on the bladder mucosa. The treatment is antibiotic therapy (sometimes long-term) aimed at the offending organism.

19.3.2.5. Metabolic Complications

Without enough patient fluid intake, acidosis and dehydration can occur from loss of salt (bicarbonate) in the urine. Treatment is with salt supplementation (bicarbonate tablets) and the administration of mineralocorticoids.

19.3.2.6. Reflux Pancreatitis

This complication presents with elevations of serum amylase and lipase. Treatment is with long-term catheterization and alpha blockade.

19.3.2.7. Bladder Mucosal Neoplasia

There are anecdotal reports of the development of neoplasia in bladder mucosa bathed with nonphysiologic pancreatic exocrine secretions.

19.3.3. Other Complications

Hypoglycemia after pancreas transplantation may occur secondary to anti-insulin antibodies or continued gastric enteropathy. In terms of surgical complications, the incidence of *incisional hernias* is the same as for other solid organ transplants.

Mortality after the initial postoperative period is most commonly secondary to myocardial infarction. In a recent 3-year follow-up study, half of the deaths occurred in the first 6 months.

Chapter 20

Results of Abdominal Organ Transplantation

David J. Reich, Jorge A. Ortiz,
and Cosme Manzarbeitia

20.1. LIVER TRANSPLANTATION

The field of liver transplantation has blossomed since the first transplants were performed in the 1960s and 1970s. Improvements in operative technique, anesthetic management, postoperative care, organ preservation solutions, and immunosuppression have contributed to marked increases in patient and graft survival rates. It should be noted that increased patient and graft survival over the past few decades comes in the face of transplanting higher risk recipients, with the use of more and more extended donor livers.

20.1.1. Overall Survival

In general, 1- and 5-year patient survival rates after liver transplantation approach 90% and 80%, respectively. One- and 5-year graft survival rates approach 85% and 75%, respectively. Graft survival rates are somewhat lower than patient survival rates because some recipients require retransplantation. Although there are morbidity and mortality from chronic immunosuppression, disease recurrence, chronic rejection, and technical problems, the major cause of mortality in recipients with long-term follow-up has become cardiovascular disease.

20.1.2.   Factors Affecting Survival

When subgroups of liver transplant recipients are studied, it becomes clear that there is a spectrum of expected survival, depending on various preoperative, intraoperative, and postoperative factors. Understanding risk factors for poor outcome after transplantation is important not only for prognostication but also to better use the scarce resource of a liver allograft.

20.1.2.1.   Preoperative Risk Factors

The liver recipient's age, severity of disease, and particular liver disease affect posttransplant survival.

20.1.2.1a. Age.   Recipients under the age of 60 fare better than those older than 60, but more and more senior citizens are receiving liver transplantation as outcomes improve. Certainly, patients with significant cardiorespiratory disease, diabetes, obesity, or other significant comorbidities, are at increased risk for complications after transplantation.

20.1.2.1b. Severity of Liver Disease.   More important than the particular age of the recipient is the severity of liver disease at the time of transplantation. Numerous studies have shown that early referral of patients with liver disease to hepatologists and liver transplant centers is a prerequisite for timely transplantation and thus improved outcome. Patients with advanced CPT scores, severe ascites (especially spontaneous bacterial peritonitis), renal failure, hypoalbuminemia, malnutrition, or advanced United Network of Organ Sharing (UNOS) scores all have increased risk for posttransplant complications. Patients on life support at the time of transplantation and those with significant infections are at highest risk for poor survival.

20.1.2.1c. Particular Liver Disease.   The particular disease for which a patient receives liver transplantation impacts on long-term survival. In recipients, large hepatocellular carcinomas (greater than 5 cm and/or more than three lesions) are prone to recurrence, and this group of patients has the least favorable survival after liver transplantation. It should be noted that patients with less extensive hepatomas, whether diagnosed preoperatively or found incidentally, are not at increased risk for posttransplant recurrence. Patients transplanted for chronic hepatitis B used to suffer a high incidence of disease recurrence and mortality. However, since the advent of lamivudine, a potent antiviral medication, survival after transplantation for hepatitis B is excellent. Patients with chronic hepatitis C also suffer recurrence, but most recurrences do not necessitate graft replacement, nor do they lead to mortality. Patients transplanted for cholestatic liver disease (biliary cirrhosis, sclerosing cholangitis) enjoy the best outcomes after liver transplantation.

Patients transplanted for fulminant hepatic failure suffer increased complications and mortality. Many of these patients are transplanted *in extremis* because of rapid disease progression. These patients have lower rates of 1-year patient (65% vs. 80%) and allograft (53% vs. 70%) survival compared to patients with nonfulminant disease. However, these differences disappear when risk is adjusted for other factors, such as postoperative ICU stay and donor status. Outcomes after liver transplantation for fulminant hepatic failure are improved if, based on prognostic criteria, transplantation is performed before the patient is moribund. This is difficult to do, because there is concern about not transplanting those that might recover without liver replacement.

20.1.2.2. Operative Risk Factors

Technically complex transplants are prone to increased intraoperative hemorrhage, necessitating multiple transfusions of packed red blood cells and other blood products. The requirement for massive transfusion is an indicator of poor outcome posttransplant.

20.1.2.2a. Prior Surgery. Recipients with a history of right-upper-quadrant surgery, such as cholecystectomy or portocaval shunt, are at increased risk for operative complications. Development of varices within thickened adhesions contributes to the technical difficulties during surgery. The extreme situation of prior liver transplantation poses particular technical difficulties, and late re-transplantation can be a *tour de force.*

20.1.2.2b. Portal Vein Thrombosis. Portal vein thrombosis used to be an absolute contraindication to liver transplantation, but patients with this complication are currently transplanted using venous jump grafts to patent mesenteric veins. In the face of complete mesenteric venous thrombosis, transplantation may be possible using cavoportal hemitransposition; in such cases, the donor portal vein receives inflow from the recipient vena cava.

20.1.2.2c. Obesity. Patients with chronic liver disease and malnutrition can still suffer obesity. Transplantation of obese, and even morbidly obese, recipients is on the rise and poses technical difficulties.

20.1.2.3. Postoperative Risk Factors

Postoperative factors that contribute to decreased patient and/or graft survival included poor early graft function, primary nonfunction, sepsis, and technical complications such as hepatic artery thrombosis or bile leak. Patients with long-term follow-up also suffer morbidity and/or mortality from disease recurrence, chronic rejection, and the side effects of chronic immunosuppression. Recipients with long-term follow-up are more likely to die from cardiovascular disease than from complications directly related to transplantation or liver disease.

20.1.3. Quality of Life

Most liver transplant recipients enjoy an excellent quality of life in the long term. During the first year, posttransplant recipients reduce their medication requirements, so that most require only a few pills per day. Healthy recipients with long-term follow-up require doctor visits and blood work only a few times a year. Most recipients are fit, psychologically well off, and perform routine activities of daily living, including employment or running a household.

20.1.4. Pregnancy after Liver Transplantation

Women may safely bear children after liver transplantation. Although there is more to be learned about the teratogenic effects of various immunosuppressants, many children have been born to mothers taking cyclosporine or tacrolimus, and the incidence of complications has been relatively low. Transplant recipients have a small, increased risk of giving birth to premature and/or gestationally small-for-age children. Recipients that suffer allograft rejection during pregnancy are at particularly high risk for fetal as well as maternal complications. Therefore, it is recommended that women wait approximately 1 to 2 years posttransplant before attempting conception, so that they are fully recovered from the transplant, are maintained adequately on low levels of immunosuppression, and are past the period of significant risk of rejection. Liver transplant recipients may deliver vaginally or via caesarean section.

20.2. KIDNEY TRANSPLANTATION

There are ample data on survival and results after kidney transplantation. This data can be studied from different perspectives, depending on the goals desired in reporting. Most centers report both patient and graft survival at 1, 3, and 5 years. As a general indicator of results, the overall 1-year patient and graft survival rates are high, generally above 80%. However, results vary depending on the cohort or factors studied. Living donor kidney transplantation is superior to cadaveric renal transplantation. The graft and patient survival rates for recipients of cadaveric donor kidneys are 88% and 95% at 1 year, and 72% and 88% at 3 years, respectively. In comparison, the living donor graft and patient survival rates are 95% and 98% at 1 year, and 85% and 95% at 3 years, respectively. The half-life of a kidney from a live donor transplanted in 1996 is 16.7 years as opposed to that of a cadaveric renal allograft, which is 10.4 years. In living related renal transplantation, the operation is planned; waiting time is frequently about 2 to 3 months; the incidence of delayed function is greatly reduced and more cost-effective than dialysis or cadaveric donor transplantation.

Results also vary according to disease etiology, but these variations are small, with most graft survival rates at about 88 to 95%, depending on the origin of the graft. Worse results are seen in highly sensitized patients, such as those with panel reactive antibody percentage (PRA) > 80%, whose cadaveric donor graft survival approaches 80%. Also, if the renal allograft required dialysis support within the first week posttransplant, graft survival can drop to the 65–75% range. All of these data have both medical and economical implications. Overall, results have been improving due mostly to better immunosuppressive agents and antibiotics. Patient survival is invariably higher than graft survival, due to the availability of dialysis support after the graft fails.

The human leukocyte antigen (HLA) matching of kidneys has received much attention in the past as an indicator of graft survival. However, the experience in living donors, showing little difference in results in anything less than HLA-identical siblings, has brought to light the fact that the really important factors are donor health and short cold-ischemic time. These data have yet to be reflected in the kidney allocation system.

20.3. PANCREAS TRANSPLANTATION

Pancreas transplantation is a procedure offered to diabetic patients, usually with associated end-stage kidney disease. The results of this type of procedure have improved over the years. As mentioned in Chapter 12, pancreas transplantation can be performed simultaneously with a kidney transplant (SPK), after a previous kidney transplant (PAK), or alone, without kidney transplantation (PTA). The best results, with a patient 1-year survival rate of over 90% and a graft 1-year survival rate of over 80%, are obtained with SPK. Pancreas graft survival for PAK is significantly less than with SPK, and current 1-year graft survival rates for PTA stand at 52%.

20.3.1. Graft Loss and Immunosuppression

Rejection accounts for 32% of graft failures in the first year after transplantation. Standard immunosuppression for pancreas transplantation has undergone an evolution similar to that for kidney transplantation. Quadruple therapy with cyclosporine, steroids, OKT3, and azathioprine gave way to quadruple therapy with tacrolimus, steroids, IL-2 inhibitors, and mycophenolate. Some centers employ different variations on these themes, including the use of bone marrow, sirolimus, and steroid-free regimens. Simultaneous bone marrow infusion with triple immunosuppression was reported by the University of Pittsburgh to result in a higher steroid withdrawal rate, fewer rejection episodes, and no graft loss secondary to chronic rejection (*Annals of Surgery* 1999;*230*,3:372–381). The University of Pittsburgh (*Transplantation* 2000;*69*,2:265–271) and the University of Minnesota (*Clinical Transplants* 2000;*14*,1:75–78) have published data advocating the use of tacrolimus and steroids in the immediate postoperative period, with withdrawal of steroids at 1 year.

20.3.2. Survival Rates and Results

Long-term survival for Type 1 diabetics on dialysis and Type 1 diabetic kidney transplant recipients is dismal. The 1-year survival for 2,387 SPKs performed in the United States between 1994–1997 is 82%. Tyden et al. (*Transplantation* 1999;*67*,5:645–648) reported 80% 10-year survival rate of Type 1 diabetics with functioning pancreas grafts compared with a 20% 10-year survival in Type 1 diabetics who only had functioning kidney grafts. The University of Wisconsin reported the world's largest experience with pancreas transplantation. Patient 1-, 5-, and 10-year survival rates were 96.4%, 88.6%, and 76.3%, respectively. Kidney graft survival rates were 88.6%, 80.3%, and 66.6%, respectively. Pancreas function rates over the same time period were 87.5%, 78.1%, and 67.2%, respectively (*Annals of Surgery* 1998;*228*,3:284–296).

The purpose of pancreas transplantation is to arrest or improve secondary diabetic complications, which, we hope, would lead to greater patient survival and enhanced quality of life. The recurrence of *diabetic nephropathy* in diabetic patients who receive only a kidney is well known. There has been documented histologic improvement in native kidneys after pancreas transplant alone. After SPK, long-term kidney survival is equivalent to kidney survival in the nondiabetic patient. After 3 years with a functioning pancreatic graft, *diabetic retinopathy* stabilizes. Symptomatic improvement and measurable increase in both nerve conduction and sensory action potentials have followed successful pancreas transplantation. Diabetic gastroparesis also improves. There is less pronounced progression in carotid lesions in pancreas recipients compared to those who have never received a transplant. In terms of lipid profiles, high-density lipoprotein (HDL) cholesterol increases while total cholesterol and triglyceride levels decrease, and left ventricular function appears to improve to a greater degree after successful pancreas transplantation when compared to kidney transplantation alone.

In terms of *quality of life*, patients report more positive perceptions of health, less pain, and greater ability to function socially. Additionally, pancreas and kidney transplantations can restore fertility in uremic patients. Occasional graft losses and congenital malformations have been noted in the birthing period. As for the *economic aspects*, the estimated annual medical expenditures for diabetes care and management in pancreas transplant candidates are about $10,000–$15,000 a year. The average annual cost of dialysis is roughly $45,000 a year. After 5 years with a functioning graft, pancreas transplantation becomes cost-effective.

Data show that pancreas transplantation leads to extended long-term survival, improvement of secondary complications of diabetes, and enhanced quality of life. Improved immunosuppression, better surgical techniques, and procurement solutions promise to yield continued success in the coming years.

Part VI

Diagnostic Tools in Abdominal Transplantation

Chapter **21**

Pathology of Transplantation
Nayere Zaeri and Ierachmiel Daskal

The transplant professional counts heavily on the contributions of the pathologist for diagnosis before and after transplantation. While it is not the purpose of this manual to offer a description of all the conditions that lead to end-stage organ disease, it is important to offer an overview of posttransplant pathology as it pertains to diagnosis and management of acute rejection and other conditions that cause allograft dysfunction in the postoperative period. Finally, due to the sparse and often controversial information regarding pancreatic allograft biopsies, only liver and kidney transplantation are addressed here.

21.1. LIVER TRANSPLANT

The spectrum of liver transplant pathology begins with the *examination of the recipient's explanted liver*. This is a valuable opportunity to study the primary disease in depth and to search carefully for other pathologic features, such as incidental hepatocellular carcinoma.

The *donor liver* can be evaluated rapidly before transplantation. Frozen-section technique is usually used for such an examination. The presence and the degree of steatosis (most importantly, macrovesicular steatosis), inflammation, necrosis, and fibrosis can be evaluated immediately by this technique. The liver with severe macrovesicular steatosis, usually involving more than 30% of parenchyma is at high risk for early graft failure (Fig. 21.1).

At the *time of transplantation*, a postperfusion liver biopsy (0 time) can be utilized to estimate the degree of preservation injury. The peak of morphologic changes, however, occurs after 48 hours, when centrizonal hepatocellular swelling

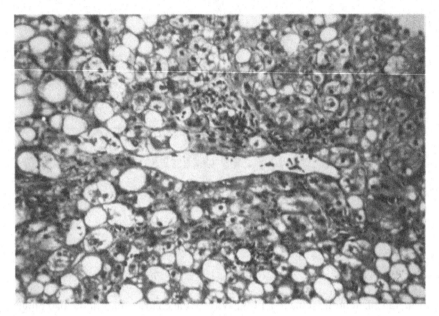

Figure 21.1. Severe macrovesicular steatosis involving more than 30% of hepatocytes (Trichome stain).

and cholestasis can be appreciated. The liver with a significant degree of macrovesicular steatosis is more susceptible to perfusion injury and a higher incidence of early graft failure.

After transplantation, monitoring of the hepatic functions and histopathologic examination of the allograft remain the most reliable methods for posttransplant management. The major causes of early allograft dysfunction are acute rejection, mechanical or technical complications, and infections. *Acute graft rejection* generally develops between 1 and 3 weeks posttransplant. Late acute graft rejection is possibly due to changes in immunosuppression regimen. Needle biopsy is used for accurate diagnosis of acute rejection. Fine-needle aspirate, although not widely accepted, has also been used in some transplant centers. Bile duct epithelium and blood vessels are the major targets of rejection. The three major diagnostic features are (1) mixed but predominantly lymphocytic portal infiltrate, (2) bile duct injury, and (3) endotheliatitis (Fig. 21.2). The portal infiltrate is composed of activated lymphocytes, polymorphonuclear leukocytes, and eosinophils. The bile duct epithelium shows nuclear crowding, cytoplasmic vacuolization, enlarged nuclei, and prominent nucleoli. Endothelialitis consists of inflammatory infiltrate of the vessel wall, usually the portal vein, but sometimes the terminal venule, associated with endothelial cell swelling and separation.

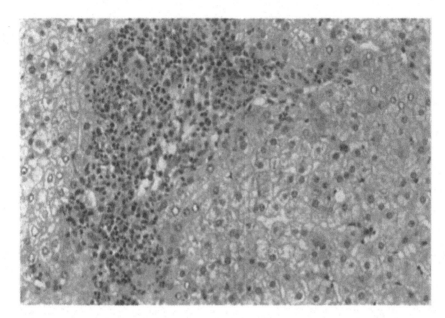

Figure 21.2. Acute cellular rejection, with mixed portal infiltrate, bile duct injury, and endothelialitis (H&E stain).

Once the diagnosis of rejection is established, grading should be assessed. The most recent and widely accepted system is the Banff Consensus Schema. Grading is based upon global assessment of portal infiltrate and the rejection activity index. According to the global assessment, the rejection is mild when a few portal triads contain reduced and confined portal infiltrate, moderate when the infiltrate expands most of the portal triads, and severe when portal infiltrate extends into the periportal area, with perivenule infiltrate and hepatocyte necrosis. The rejection activity index is based on a total numerical score obtained by adding each component of rejection: portal infiltrate, bile duct inflammation, and endothelial inflammation.

Mechanical complications, usually presenting early after transplantation, include *vascular* and *bile duct complications*. Thrombosis or fibrosis of the hepatic artery or portal vein at the anastomosis site can result in ischemia of allograft. Bile duct injury, such as stricture or breakdown, can lead to biliary obstruction, peritonitis, and sepsis.

The allograft is susceptible to various opportunistic infections, particularly viral infection. *Cytomegaloviral* (CMV) *hepatitis* usually occurs in the first 2 to 3 months after transplantation. On infrequent occasions, CMV hepatitis can mimic rejection. The hallmark of histologic diagnosis is microabscesses (Fig. 21.3) with

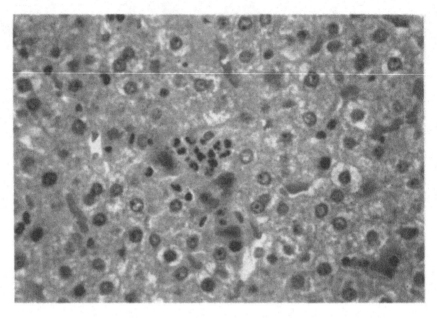

Figure 21.3. Microabscess in transplantation (cytomegalovirus).

viral inclusions (Fig. 21.4). Immunohistochemical staining can enhance the sensitivity of histologic detection.

Late allograft dysfunction, usually occurring at 3 months and beyond, encompasses several complex conditions requiring combined clinical and pathologic evaluation. *Chronic rejection*, sometimes as a result of unrecognized ongoing rejection, has less defined diagnostic–pathologic features. Histologically, chronic rejection occurs/or may be suspected when there is progressive bile duct disappearance and obliterative arteriopathy. The criterion, absence of more than 50% of interlobular bile ducts, particularly on multiple, consecutive biopsies, provides a reliable histologic feature of irreversible chronic rejection. The portal areas usually have minimal inflammatory infiltrate. Obliterative arteriopathy usually involves the larger blood vessels and is not detectable by percutaneous needle biopsy. It is characterized by collections of intimal foamy macrophages and subsequent intimal thickening and luminal obliteration.

Hepatitis B and C infections recur in 80–100% of cases. A subfulminant form of hepatitis B, known as fibrosing cholestatic hepatitis, can occur and carries a bad prognosis. End-stage liver disease due to hepatitis C is now the major cause for liver transplant in the United States. Recurrent hepatitis C has overlapping features with rejection and, therefore, may require clinical–pathologic correlation to reach the specific diagnosis. Portal infiltrate with lymphocytic preponderance, bile

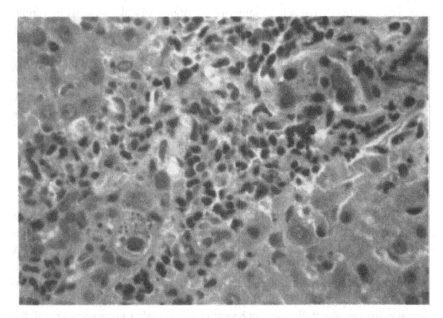

Figure 21.4. Viral inclusions with cytopathic effect (cytomegalovirus).

duct inflammatory changes, and lobular inflammation are constant features of recurrent hepatitis C. Predominant lobular hepatitis and liver cell necrosis (apoptotic liver cells) are features in favor of recurrent hepatitis C. Other recurrent diseases have been described (although not widely accepted) in allografts: primary biliary cirrhosis, primary sclerosing cholangitis, and autoimmune disease. Rarely, recurrent malignant neoplasm can affect the allograft.

Posttransplant lymphoproliferative disorder (PTLD), an Epstein–Barr virus (EBV)-related complication, usually occur later after transplantation. The most serious of all PTLDs is monoclonal B-cell lymphoma.

Finally, late hepatic allograft dysfunction can be caused by *drug-induced liver injury*. These patients are often on multiple medications, and either toxicity or drug interactions can cause elevation of liver enzymes and histopathologic changes. Therefore, it is important to interpret the liver biopsies of these patients with knowledge of their medications and immunosuppression levels.

21.2. KIDNEY TRANSPLANT

Renal allograft loss following transplantation can be attributed to a large number of factors, both immune and nonimmune. The nonimmune factors may consist of perfusion (ischemic) injury of the organ, vascular stenosis of various etiologies (surgical, thrombotic, infectious), various bacterial and viral infections, cyclosporine (CyA), tacrolimus (FK506), monoclonal antibody (OKT3) related toxicities, recurrence of primary renal disease (diabetes, uncontrolled hypertension, etc.), and *de novo* glomerular diseases. Last but not least, immunosuppression-induced PTLD may be included in this list. It is beyond the scope of this manual to discuss these factors in any detail; only a few of the more common reasons for graft loss are mentioned briefly.

21.2.1. Organ Selection

One of the most important roles of the transplant pathologist is to evaluate an organ for its suitability for transplantation and its postperfusion status. This assessment must take place prior to and immediately after transplantation. A small-needle biopsy is submitted for frozen-section evaluation. Commonly encountered problems consist of glomerular obsolescence (sclerosis), disseminated intravascular coagulation (DIC), thrombosis, interstitial fibrosis, advanced hypertensive disease, silent diabetic nephropathy, or any other unsuspected renal disease. Progressive glomerular sclerosis and obsolescence have been associated with poor graft survival. Kidneys that have in excess of 20% sclerotic glomeruli should be rejected for transplantation, since about 90% of such kidneys developed delayed graft function and about 38% of the grafts were lost. Immediately following transplantation another histopathological assessment should take place to determine proper organ perfusion as well as the extent of acute tubular necrosis (ATN), if present. This evaluation should be made on permanent sections. The findings must be communicated to the surgeon immediately.

21.2.2. Immune-Mediated Rejection

21.2.2.1. Hyperacute Rejection

21.2.2.1a. Clinical.   Hyperacute rejection in an organ occurs in the very first minutes to hours postrevascularization. Instead of assuming a bright pinkish-red color following perfusion, the organ immediately turns dusky and dark. The kidney is edematous and enlarged secondary to congestion. It is nonfunctional and does not produce urine.

21.2.2.1b. Histopathology.   The humoral arm of the immune system mediates hyperacute rejection. It occurs when there is a major blood group incompatibility and/or a major human leukocyte antigen (HLA) Class I mismatch.

Circulating antibodies bind to endothelial cells surfaces, activate the coagulation system, and initiate thrombosis. The presence of neutrophils within glomeruli and peritubular capillaries is a common diagnostic feature in the very early phase of hyperacute rejection. Extensive interstitial edema and hemorrhage accompanied by vascular thrombosis are present. Within the glomeruli, there is significant red blood cell (RBC) congestion and infiltration of neutrophils. At more advanced stages, within 12–24 hours, frank cortical necrosis may be present. Tubular epithelial necrosis is seen as well. Immunofluorescent studies on such kidneys reveal an intense anti-IgM and -C3 antigen staining of the deposits within the vascular and glomerular lesions.

21.2.2.2. Acute Humoral Rejection

This form of rejection can occur within the first 3–4 months posttransplant. It is also mediated by the humoral immune system. Similar to hyperacute rejection, this process is also mediated by anti-HLA Class I antibodies. The histological picture is that of thrombotic microangiopathy, involving both glomeruli and arterioles. Immunofluorescence of anti-C4d complement fraction in peritubular capillaries is diagnostic. Fibrinoid necrosis of arterioles, which may be present in 25% of cases, confers a poor prognosis for graft survival. Recovery is only about 50–60%. The major differential diagnosis is that of CyA toxicity.

21.2.2.3. Acute Vascular Rejection

An intense transmural-necrotizing lesion may be seen in larger arteries. It consists of medial myocyte necrosis with fibrin deposition within the media of arterioles. Immunofluorescence shows anti-IgM, -IgG, -C3, and fibrin deposition. This lesion indicates a very poor prognosis for graft survival and is also mediated by the humoral immune system.

21.2.2.4. Acute Cellular Rejection

21.2.2.4a. Clinical.   Acute cellular rejection (ACR) can occur within the first week up to years posttransplantation. It is manifested clinically by a rise in serum creatinine, which may be subtle and gradual or quite sudden.

21.2.2.4b. Histopathology.   The cellular arm of the immune system mediates acute cellular rejection. Each renal compartment exhibits characteristic features in ACR. Commonly, these consist of an inflammatory cell infiltrate composed of activated T cells of variable intensity. This infiltrate frequently targets endothelial cells, tubular epithelium, and interstitium of the kidney.

The characteristic feature of ACR in the glomerulus is the presence of luminal mononuclear cells within the capillaries. Because the endothelium is among the first cells to express donor antigens, the host T cells are seen to attach to it. This phenomenon is known as posttransplant glomerulitis (PTG). It is seen frequently in the immediate period posttransplantation and may be a part of the broader constellation of ACR. Commonly, PTG is seen in the first 4–6 weeks posttransplantation.

The classical manifestation of ACR in the tubular epithelial cells is the infiltration of lymphocytes into at least 5% of the cortical tubular epithelial cells, a phenomenon known as tubulitis. The infiltrating lymphocytes can be identified by the small, clear "halo" that surrounds them. Rejection-type tubulitis must be differentiated from "senile tubulitis," present in atrophic tubules, which is the final common pathway of tubular destruction regardless of etiology. Multiple fields and levels of sections containing cortical tissue should be examined to determine the extent of tubulitis.

Similarly, an interstitial inflammatory cell infiltrate is commonly seen in ACR. It is composed primarily of activated T cells, predominantly CD8(+). Subcapsular infiltrates should be excluded from the consideration for ACR. Occasionally, neutrophils and eosinophils may be present as well. This infiltrate may be focal and intense at times.

The activated T cells home in on the vascular endothelium, a major antigenic presentation site in ACR. As such, the T cells will adhere within the luminal endothelial cells or may be seen infiltrating underneath the endothelial layer of arteries and arterioles. This is known as vasculitis, endothelialitis, or endarteritis. In more severe ACR cases, medium-size and larger arterioles may be involved. Transmural infiltration of lymphocytes or a frank necrotizing arteritis can be seen in severe cases of rejection and frequently lead to organ loss. There are no significant diagnostic immunofluorescence findings in ACR.

21.2.2.4c. Differential Diagnosis for Acute Cellular Rejection. CyA toxicity may resemble ACR. Tubulitis may be present but is the hallmark of ACR, not CyA toxicity. The main target of drug toxicity is the proximal convoluted tubules. An important feature of acute CyA toxicity is the presence of numerous minute vacuoles within the tubular cells, known as "isometric vacuolation." Unlike ACR, there is no evidence for an interstitial mononuclear cell infiltrate in CyA toxicity. In acute tubulointerstitial rejection, there is a diffuse lymphocytic infiltrate. A sparser infiltrate is present in CyA toxicity. Thrombotic microangiopathy, similar to that seen in acute humoral rejection, may be seen with CyA toxicity. This cannot be differentiated from microangiopathy of other etiologies.

PTLD should also be considered in the differential diagnosis. The presence of large number of activated B cells instead of T cells would suggest the presence of PTLD rather than ACR. An intense infiltrate of eosinophils and basophils may be seen in acute drug toxicity. An acute interstial nephritis of infectious or reactive etiologies can be difficult to differentiate from ACR. An infectious etiology for the process should be ruled out (polyoma [BK virus], EBV, CMV).

21.2.2.5. Chronic Rejection

21.2.2.5a. Clinical. Chronic rejection can be seen from months to years after transplantation and is a common cause for graft loss. A gradual deterioration of renal function is commonly seen. A biopsy is recommended to document rejection.

21.2.2.5b. Histopathology. The tubules and interstitium show increased interstitial fibrosis and tubular atrophy, with a mononuclear cell infiltrate. Tubular basement membranes are thickened and duplicated. An acute cellular rejection process may also coexist with this chronic process. It is believed that the tubular lesion in chronic graft rejection is mediated by increased ischemia (see vascular lesions below) and repeated bouts of ACR.

Within the glomeruli, there is evidence for mesangial expansion and, especially, duplication and webbing of capillary basement membranes. Known as "transplant glomerulopathy," this must be differentiated from hepatitis C virus (HCV) nephropathy and other membranoproliferative glomerulonephritis (GN) of other etiologies. A thrombotic microangiopathic picture, similar to that noted in CyA toxicity, may be seen as well. Focal or global sclerosis of glomeruli may be present. At times a glomerular tip lesion may develop. This consists of the adhesion of a glomerular capillary to the origin of the proximal convoluted tubule. It is believed that the transplant glomerulopathy is the result of immune attack on the endothelial cells of the glomerulus.

Within vessels, the characteristic lesion of chronic rejection consists of intimal proliferation and fibrous thickening, with infiltration of foamy macrophages within the media. A subendothelial mononuclear cell infiltrate is often present. The pathogenesis of the chronic arterial lesion appears at present to be multifactorial. Immunofluorescent studies in chronic allograft rejection are nonspecific. However, these are important to exclude recurrent or *de novo* glomerular disease.

21.2.2.5c. Differential Diagnosis of Chronic Rejection. Chronic rejection may not be differentiated for chronic CyA or FK506 toxicity. The presence of transplant glomerulopathy or "webbing" is not seed in CyA toxicity. Chronic transplant glomerulopathy must be differentiated from HCV or other membranoproliferative glomerulonephropathy. Immunofluorescence (IFE) may be important to determine whether *de novo* immune complex glomerulonephropathy is present. Interstitial fibrosis caused by chronic rejection cannot be readily differentiated from CyA toxicity. Large lymphocytic infiltrates, composed primarily of B lymphocytes are more likely to represent PTLD than chronic rejection. Subintimal hyaliosis, seen in benign hypertension, should not be confused with the presence of intimal fibrin seen in chronic rejection.

21.2.3. Scoring Rejection

The most current approach for scoring rejection was developed by an expert panel of pathologists, in lieu of the previous Banff classification, first proposed in 1993. Sponsored by the National Institutes of Health (NIH), the Cooperative Clinical Trials in Transplantation (CCTT), defined three main categories in acute rejection.

- *Type I*—ACR, primarily representing tubulointerstial rejection. This is frequently responsive to steroid therapy.
- *Type II*—ACR more severe than Type I and represented primarily by the presence of endarteritis.
- *Type III*—the most severe ACR, with the poorest prognosis for graft survival. It is represented by transmural inflammation and vascular fibrinoid necrosis of arterioles and arteries. Several retrospective studies have confirmed the reproducibility of this schema.

21.2.4. Immunosuppressive Drug Toxicity

One of the most common adverse effects of CyA treatment is toxicity that may lead to graft loss. Three major categories of CyA nephrotoxicity exist: acute toxicity, chronic toxicity, and thrombotic microangiopathy. Some of the more acute changes, such as isometric vacuolation of the proximal convoluted tubules, were addressed earlier.

Tubular atrophy, present in *chronic CyA toxicity*, frequently presents in a segmental manner, yielding a "stripped" pattern. This will occur from a few months to years following transplantation and depends largely on the history of drug administration. The characteristic chronic lesion is an induced arteriopathy, which consists primarily of single myocyte degeneration. Later, hyaline–fibrin replace the necrotic myocytes within the media in a pearl-like or beaded form. This may appear as a proteinaceous deposit on the outer periphery of the affected vessels, leaving the intimal layer intact. The external nodular hyalinosis may also be seen in other disorders but with less frequency than that of CyA toxicity. This should be differentiated from the subintimal hyalinosis seen in diabetes and benign hypertension.

Thrombotic microangiopathy, similar to that present in acute humoral rejection, may be seen in high-dose CyA toxicity. Renal failure, increased lactate dehydrogenase (LDH) levels, and hemolytic anemia may accompany thrombotic microangiopathy. Most of the toxic side effects of FK506 are similar to those of CyA. Administration of prophylactic OKT3 10 mg/day for 2 weeks induced an increased rate of glomerular thrombosis (microangiopathic type). Thrombosis of major arteries was found as well.

21.2.5. Posttransplantation Lymphoproliferative Disorders (PTLDs)

PTLD tends to occur as early as 6 weeks postinitiation of immunosuppressive therapy, with incidence of 1–2% of all transplants. It is believed that EBV mediates it, either as an epiphenomenon or as a direct cause. The most common clinical presentation is a gradual loss of graft function. The histopathology consists of a dense, massive infiltrate of B-type lymphocytes, some with some plasmacytic differentiation, which may be mono- or polyclonal. Immunohistochemical studies as well as *in situ* hybridization are useful in detecting EBV components within the lesion. Once diagnosed, patient are managed with dose reduction or temporary stoppage of immunosuppressive therapy.

21.2.6. Other Causes for Graft Loss

21.2.6.1. Ischemic Injury

Frequently, cold preservation of kidneys prior to transplantation causes acute ischemic injury to the tubular epithelial cells. This lesion is believed to cause delayed graft function. The histological spectrum of this lesion ranges from excessively large vacuolation of tubular cells to loss of brush border of proximal convoluted tubules, to individual cell necrosis.

21.2.6.2. Viral Infections

Viral infections are common in renal transplant patients. Among the more common ones is CMV, which can cause graft loss and may simulate rejection. EBV is presently implicated in PTLD and BK (polyoma) virus, which can also cause graft loss. HCV infection is seen in approximately 10% of patients and has been associated with increased risk of acute graft glomerulopathy. Histologically, this lesion is similar to membranoproliferative glomerulonephritis (MPGN) and hence must be differentiated from it as well as from chronic transplant glomerulopathy. Occurring less frequently are infections caused by human herpes viruses

(HHV 1, 2, and 6) and adenoviruses. Molecular and immunohistochemical techniques readily differentiate between these viruses.

21.2.6.3. De Novo *Glomerulonephritis*

Transplanted patients without prior history of glomerular disease may develop lesions that clinically may simulate rejection. Membranous glomerulonephritis (MGN) may be seen in 2% of transplants anywhere from 2 months to 5 years after transplantation, with an average of approximately 2 years. It appears that the epimembranous deposits in transplanted MGN are somewhat smaller than those in idiopathic MGN. It is believed that the etiology of transplant MGN is antibodies that work against minor histocompatibility sites.

21.2.6.4. *Other* De Novo *Glomerulopathies*

Occurring less frequently are antiglomerular basement membrane (anti-GBM) glomerulopathies and focal segmental glomerulosclerosis (FSGS). The anti-GBM lesions were seen in grafts transplanted into patients with Alport's disease. These cases commonly also develop a crescenteric glomerulonephritis. FSGS has been described primarily in adult patients who received pediatric allografts. The presumed etiology of this lesion is hyperfiltration of the transplanted kidney. Both the classical and the collapsing variant of FSGS may be seen.

21.2.6.5. *Recurrent Diseases*

Up to 5% of graft failures may be attributed to recurrent disease. The more common ones are diabetic nephropathy, dense deposit disease, FSGS, IgA nephropathy MPGN, hemolytic–uremic syndrome, Henoch–Schönlein purpura, and MGN.

Chapter 22

Radiology in Transplantation
Juan Oleaga

With the development of new and improved imaging modalities and less invasive percutaneous techniques, diagnostic and interventional radiology have an increasing and significant role in the pre- and posttransplant evaluation and management of transplant donors and recipients.

22.1. PRETRANSPLANT EVALUATION

The main role of radiological evaluation of potential donors and recipients is to determine the presence of coexistent conditions that will increase the risk of, preclude, or alter transplantation. The multimodality approach is required due to the inherent strengths and weaknesses of each technique. The precise protocol used by different centers is variable depending on local equipment and expertise.

22.1.1. Liver

The pretransplant evaluation of the liver recipient involves the following modalities:

22.1.1.1. Duplex Ultrasound

Duplex ultrasound is the least invasive and probably most used imaging modality in the pretransplant evaluation. Its safety, availability, and proven ability to evaluate the hepatic parenchyma; the patency of the portal veins, hepatic artery, hepatic veins, and inferior vena cava; and biliary ductal dilatation are valuable in patient selection; it is the initial study of choice.

22.1.1.2. Computed Tomography

Preoperative, routine computed tomography (CT) scan evaluation is useful in determining the presence of ascites, varices, and other signs of portal hypertension, liver volume, and focal or diffuse lesions. CT arterial portography has aided in detecting liver neoplasms, especially metastases. However, its usefulness in liver transplantation has been limited due to altered hepatic hemodynamics secondary to cirrhosis, and it requires placement of a selective catheter in the splenic or superior mesenteric arteries. Three-dimensional, helical CT angiography (CTA) is a noninvasive technique that is useful to evaluate the normal and variant arterial supply of the liver. The need for intravenous (IV) conventional radiographic contrast may limit the use of CT scan techniques in patients with renal insufficiency or contrast allergies.

22.1.1.3. Magnetic Resonance

Magnetic resonance imaging (MRI) and angiography (MRA) techniques have evolved rapidly and complement traditional modalities. With its tissue-specific contrast agents, multiplanar imaging, and special techniques such as chemical shift and fat suppression, MRI provides improved detection and characterization of focal liver lesions, and is excellent in diagnosing fatty infiltration of the liver and hemochromatosis. Contrast-enhanced MRI can also evaluate hepatic arterial anatomy, portal vein thrombosis, and portal hypertension. However, because MRI is contraindicated in patients with magnetically, mechanically, or electrically activated implants, its application is limited.

22.1.1.4. Conventional Angiography

Visceral angiography is usually reserved as a problem-solving tool in pretransplant liver evaluation. It is useful in delineating the arterial anatomy, and identifying and characterizing preexisting vascular disease, especially in the selection process for living related transplant donors, when noninvasive modalities such as MRA or CTA have been equivocal. As an invasive technique, it is associated with an approximately 1.7% complication rate that includes contrast reactions, puncture site hematomas, distal embolization, and catheter/guide wire-related arterial injury, among others, and it may be contraindicated in patients with renal insufficiency, coagulopathy, or conventional contrast allergy.

22.1.1.5. Scintigraphy

Hepatobiliary imaging with technetium 99m IDA (iminodiacetic acid) derivatives is valuable in diagnosing and characterizing acute and chronic biliary disease, biliary obstruction, and biliary atresia. Multiple-gated acquisition scans (MUGAs) are used to evaluate the left ventricular ejection fraction. Bone scans are useful in the workup of metastases in patients with history of hepatocellular carcinoma.

22.1.2. Kidney

The diagnostic imaging evaluation of potential renal donors has been traditionally performed with duplex ultrasound of the kidneys, intravenous urograms, and conventional arteriograms, preferably, selective renal arteriograms. However, MRA and CTA, also effective in evaluating the vascular supply of potential donor kidneys, are quickly replacing other modalities.

22.1.2.1. Duplex Ultrasound

Duplex ultrasound is a noninvasive modality that is readily available, cost-effective, and has minimal risk. It is useful in evaluating potential donor kidneys for size, hydronephrosis, radiopaque or radiolucent stones, solid or cystic masses, perirenal collections, and renal parenchymal disease.

22.1.2.2. Computed Tomography

Knowledge of the renal vascular supply is crucial for successful transplantation. Variant renal arterial anatomy has an incidence of about 40%, and about 30% of individuals have multiple renal arteries. Variant venous anatomy is also common. CTA has a sensitivity and specificity of 99.6% for main renal arteries, decreasing to 76.9% and 89.9%, respectively, for accessory arteries. It is minimally invasive and as an intrinsic advantage may identify renal calculi, but since it requires IV radiographic conventional contrast, it has limited application with renal insufficiency or radiographic contrast allergy.

22.1.2.3. Magnetic Resonance

Gadolinium-enhanced MRA, like CTA, is also minimally invasive, but it does not utilize conventional radiographic contrast and can be used in renal insufficiency. In addition, like CTA, it can detect renal lesions and venous anomalies but is less likely to identify calculi. It has a sensitivity and specificity of 71% and 95%, respectively, in detecting accessory renal arteries, and 97% and 92%, respectively, in identifying main renal arteries with 50–99% stenosis. Unfortunately, MRA is contraindicated in some patients.

22.1.2.4. Conventional Angiography

As in liver transplantation, due to alternative modalities, conventional angiography is becoming a problem-solving technique. Nevertheless, it can be performed safely and effectively on an outpatient basis with small catheters and little risk. Alternative intra-arterial contrast agents such as carbon dioxide or gadolinium can be used in patients with contraindications to conventional iodinated contrast.

22.2. POSTTRANSPLANT EVALUATION AND MANAGEMENT

Precise communication and coordination among the vascular/interventional radiologists, transplant surgeons, transplant hepatologists, and a nephrologist are absolutely necessary to ensure the best possible outcome for the patients.

22.2.1. Liver

22.2.1.1. Vascular

22.2.1.1a. Hepatic Artery Thrombosis (HAT). HAT can occur in 10–42% of pediatric and 3–10% of adult liver transplants. Duplex ultrasound is the initial study of choice, with a sensitivity of 90%. Extensive arterial collaterals can result in a false-negative result. The diagnosis is suggested on the basis of absence of flow signal in the intrahepatic and porta hepatis arteries, and a tardus parvus waveform. However, due to the spectrum of abnormalities in the vasculature, visceral arteriography should be performed to confirm the diagnosis. Surgical correction is necessary. CT scan can be used to evaluate consequences of arterial thrombosis such as hepatic infarction, biloma, and abscess formation.

22.2.1.1b. Hepatic Artery Stenosis. This condition is present in 11% of transplants, and ultrasonography is the primary modality for diagnosis. The diagnosis is made when the blood velocity is > 2–3 m/sec, with turbulent flow, or if an intrahepatic tardus parvus pattern is present. As in HAT, visceral arteriography is necessary to confirm the diagnosis. Stenoses are more commonly anastomotic but can occur at adjacent sites. If detected in the immediate postoperative period, these will require surgical repair. Percutaneous transluminal angioplasty (PTA) is useful in treating stenoses 4–6 weeks posttransplant.

22.2.1.1c. Hepatic Artery Pseudoaneurysms. These are rare after liver transplants and potentially fatal if rupture occurs. They usually occur at the arterial anastomosis. They may complicate percutaneous biopsy or biliary drainages and are then intrahepatic. Patients may present with hemobilia, hemoperitoneum or gastrointestinal bleeding, or be asymptomatic, with symptoms found incidentally during routine follow-up. Both contrast-enhanced CT and ultrasound may detect pseudoaneurysms. With ultrasound, they appear as a cystic collection with swirling and disorganized flow. Arteriography shows a well-defined saccular contrast collection with persistent opacification beyond the arterial phase. If intrahepatic, they can be embolized percutaneously with coils from the intravascular approach. Those at the arterial anastomosis require surgical revision.

22.2.1.1d. Inferior Vena Cava (IVC) Thrombosis or Stenosis. This is a rare complication occurring at the anastomosis and may result in Budd–Chiari syndrome or extremity edema. Ultrasound shows focal narrowing, with three- to fourfold increase in velocity if narrowed, or intraluminal echogenic thrombus if thrombosed. The diagnosis is confirmed by venography. Percutaneous transluminal angioplasty is the treatment of choice. The initial technical and clinical success is 92%, but the stenosis is often recurrent, requiring reintervention.

22.2.1.1e. Portal Vein Complications. These are also rare, with an incidence rate of 1–13%. Symptoms are usually those of portal hypertension or hepatic failure. *Stenosis* occurs at the porta hepatis anastomosis. Ultrasound reveals an increased velocity similar to that of an IVC stenosis. If thrombosed, it will show echogenic material. If *completely thrombosed*, there will be no flow, although some flow can be detected if collaterals have developed. Angiography is best performed via the superior mesenteric artery with intra-arterial vasodilators and imaging into the venous phase. Venous thrombosis and arterial stenoses and occlusions can also be shown by MRA. The treatment of choice for portal vein stenosis is PTA via transhepatic approach. Thrombosis is best managed surgically. Percutaneous thrombolysis and stent placement may be possible.

22.2.1.2. Biliary

Biliary complications can be seen in 12–38% of liver transplant patients.

22.2.1.2a. Bile Leakage. This complication is the most common originating from the T-tube site, choledochocholedochostomy, or choledochojejunostomy. Leaks at sites other than the T-tube insertion or biliary anastomosis may be associated with arterial thrombosis. Patients may present with signs of infection or abnormally elevated bilirubin or liver enzymes. If placed operatively, a T-tube cholangiogram is the best way to evaluate the biliary tree for leaks. Preprocedure antibiotics are given, and contrast is injected by gravity drip. Ultrasound and CT scan may identify indirect evidence of a leak, such as fluid collection that could represent a biloma, and may be used as guidance for percutaneous diagnostic needle aspiration or therapeutic drainage. If a T tube is not present, hepatobiliary imaging with technetium 99m IDA derivatives is useful in detecting bile leaks by showing extraluminal radionuclide. If the cause of the biliary leak is arterial thrombosis, diversion and external drainage are a temporary solution and re-transplantation is required. However, many bile leaks may also be managed nonsurgically by draining the biloma percutaneously and diverting bile flow by opening the T tube to external drainage, repositioning the T tube, placing a percutaneous biliary drainage catheter, or endoscopically by placing a nasobiliary tube or stent. Prolonged drainage is required, since leaks may take 1 to 2 months to heal.

22.2.1.2b. Anastomotic and Nonanastomotic Biliary Strictures. These are relatively common, occurring in 4–17% of grafts. *Anastomotic strictures*, which result from scarring at the suture line, are probably the result of a technical factor, although ischemia could be a contributing factor, and are more commonly seen in patients with sclerosing cholangitis. *Nonanastomotic strictures* result from bile duct ischemia due to arterial insufficiency caused by hepatic artery stenosis or thrombosis, and may be hilar or intrahepatic. However, other causes include prolonged cold ischemia, chronic ductopenic rejection, ABO blood type incompatibility, infection, and sclerosing cholangitis. CT scan and ultrasound can reveal biliary ductal dilatation associated with strictures. Cholangiography, whether retrograde, endoscopic, or antegrade via direct transhepatic or T-tube route, is most accurate in depicting the extent and location of strictures. However, magnetic resonance cholangiography (MRC) is increasingly able to depict and detect stenoses and occlusions, although it may overestimate the degree of narrowing. Simple anastomotic strictures, whether endoscopic or percutaneous, can be treated by cholangioplasty and stenting. The stent is usually required for extended periods of 6 months or more.

22.2.1.2c. Biliary Obstruction. Several causes of biliary obstruction may complicate liver transplantation. Intrahepatic and extrahepatic stones can be readily diagnosed with ultrasound, cholangiography, or MRC. Small stones can be removed endoscopically. Larger stones can be removed percutaneously in staged procedures or surgically. Strictures can be treated with cholangioplasty, as described earlier. Rarely, obstruction can result from a cystic duct remnant mucocele that can be suggested by CT scan and ultrasound but may require needle aspiration for diagnosis. Therapy of choice is surgery.

22.2.1.3. Rejection

Currently, there are no reliable, noninvasive tests to diagnose organ rejection. Graft biopsy and histological examination remain the standard. Biopsies are performed percutaneously via the transabdominal approach using ultrasound guidance. In patients with severe ascites, coagulopathy, or thrombocytopenia as contraindications for transabdominal biopsy, a transjugular liver biopsy approach is a safe and effective alternative even in the early postoperative period.

22.2.2. Kidney

22.2.2.1. Vascular

22.2.2.1a. Renal Artery Stenosis. This can be present in up to 10% of transplant patients. Early stenosis at the anastomosis is probably a technical problem. Later, distal stenoses could result from rejection or turbulence and may present as hypertension. Ultrasound is a noninvasive modality useful in screening for arterial stenosis. Specific Doppler criteria, such as increased velocity, velocity gradients, and spectral broadening, have been developed. Scintigraphy can also be used to diagnose arterial stenosis. Findings are similar to chronic rejection except when performed with angiotensin-converting enzyme inhibitors, when the condition resembles renal artery stenosis in native kidneys. MRA can also accurately depict stenoses. A conventional arteriogram can then be performed. Carbon dioxide angiography is an alternative for patients with renal insufficiency or contrast allergy. Stenoses should be treated with percutaneous angioplasty, with surgery for recurrent stenoses. Percutaneous intravascular stent placement is another option.

22.2.2.1b. Renal Artery Thrombosis. This is rare and present in < 1% of patients. Ultrasound shows no intrarenal arterial and venous flow. Magnetic resonance can identify parenchymal areas of necrosis and absence of flow in the vessel. Findings can be confirmed with angiography. Surgical exploration is indicated.

22.2.2.1c. Renal Vein Stenosis. This condition is rare. It may result from perivascular fibrosis or compression from adjacent collection. Sonography shows increased velocities similar to arterial stenosis. Venography can be performed, if necessary, to confirm the diagnosis.

22.2.2.1d. Renal Vein Thrombosis. More common in diabetics, renal vein thrombosis may be related to cyclosporine use, presenting within a week after transplant as oliguria and an enlarged, painful kidney. Ultrasound shows an enlarged kidney with a reversed diastolic arterial waveform and absent venous flow. Thrombus may be identified in an enlarged vein. MRI shows an enlarged kidney with areas of infarction, lack of enhancement on MRA, and nonvisualization of the renal vein. A surgical thrombectomy may sometimes be possible.

22.2.2.1e. Pseudoaneurysms and Arteriovenous (AV) Fistulas. These can result from surgical technique, percutaneous biopsy, or infection. Small intrarenal pseudoaneurysms may resolve spontaneously. Larger lesions can cause ischemia, hematuria, or hemoperitoneum. Pseudoaneurysms mimic a cyst on ultrasound and have disorganized flow. AV fistulas in ultrasonography have a feeding artery with a high-velocity, low resistance waveform and a pulsatile draining vein. Intraparenchymal pseudoaneurysms may be embolized percutaneously.

22.2.2.2. Nonvascular

22.2.2.2a. Ureteric Leak and Obstruction. These are the two principal urologic complications of renal transplants. *Obstruction* early posttransplant is usually secondary to twisting of the ureter or a technical problem at the ureter implantation site. It may also result from extrinsic ureteric compression from adjacent fluid collections. Obstruction late after transplantation is probably secondary to a ureteric stricture resulting from an ischemic damage. Patients may present with oliguria and worsening renal function. Ultrasonography suggests the diagnosis by demonstrating dilated calyces and sometimes a dilated ureter. Echogenic material in the collecting system could represent infection, clots, or stones. An antegrade pyelogram may be required to confirm the diagnosis. Preprocedure antibiotics must always be given, and ultrasound guidance facilitates access. *Strictures* can be treated by balloon dilatation and stent placement either from the percutaneous antegrade or endoscopic retrograde approach. With the percutaneous approach, results are best when treating obstruction within 3 months of transplantation. Surgical revision may be required. Urine *leaks* are more common at the distal ureter and may present as fever, pain, oliguria, or wound discharge. Ultrasound and antegrade or retrograde pyelogram will establish the diagnosis. Anechoic or hypoechoic collections will be present per sonography. Pyelogram will show diffuse or contained extraluminal contrast. Scintigraphy can also show radiotracer in unusual areas. Treatment is the same as that for ureteral obstruction with placement of stents. Percutaneous drainage of focal urine collections must also be performed simultaneously.

22.2.2.2b. Perinephric Fluid Collections. Lymphoceles, urinomas, seromas, abscesses, and hematomas may complicate renal transplants. Although their appearance is nonspecific, some features may suggest their diagnosis. Lymphoceles have an incidence rate of around 5%. Their appearance in ultrasound and MRI is that of a simple fluid collection that may contain septations similar to urinomas. Lymphoceles' creatinine concentration may be similar to that of serum, which can be used to differentiate them from urinomas. Most are small, but large lymphoceles can cause mass effects on adjacent structures, such as the ureter, and result in obstruction. Percutaneous transcatheter sclerotherapy with povidone-iodine, alcohol, or bleomycin has been successful. Surgery may be required. Hematomas are easily diagnosed with MRI on the basis of their characteristic appearance on different pulse sequences.

22.2.2.2c. Diminished Renal Function. There are multiple causes of diminished renal function. Transplants affected by *hyperacute rejection* fail within minutes, are usually removed immediately, and are rarely imaged. *Acute rejection* (AR) typically occurs 1 to 3 weeks after transplantation and is present in 40–50% of transplants with chronic rejection (CR) occurring 3 months after transplantation. *Acute tubular necrosis* (ATN) may result from prolonged ischemia and typically appears within the first week, gradually resolving over 2 weeks. Clinical evolution and serial imaging studies are important in differentiating among these entities. Radionuclide scan findings for ATN and AR are similar: marked parenchymal retention and, in severe cases, no excretion into the bladder. They can be separated by their time course. ATN is present in the baseline study and improves over 2 weeks; AR rarely develops in the first week and function deteriorates on serial studies. In *chronic rejection* (CR), the renal cortex is thinned and there is mild hydronephrosis. There is decreased uptake, normal parenchymal transit, and absent/minimal cortical retention. *Cyclosporine toxicity* resembles rejection on radionuclide imaging studies. Differentiation is best with cyclosporine level and clinical correlation and serial studies. Ultrasound and MRI have not been reliable in differentiating among types of diminished renal function.

22.2.3. Pancreas

The radiologist's main role in pancreas transplant is in the diagnosis, and to a lesser extent, management of postoperative complications.

22.2.3.1. Vascular Thrombosis

The incidence rate of pancreas graft thrombosis (arterial and venous) is 5–14%, with venous thrombosis rates of 5%. Differences in the clinical presentation of patients with arterial versus venous thrombosis may suggest the diagnosis. Gadolinium-enhanced MRA is sensitive for detecting vascular compromise. Ultrasound is sensitive and specific in diagnosing venous thrombosis, using as criteria the absence of venous flow and a resistive index ≥ 1. CT angiography or selective conventional arteriography can also be used and may be necessary for diagnosis.

22.2.3.2. Rejection

Ultrasound has not been reliable in the diagnosis of graft rejection. MR can identify grafts with infarction and is sensitive for detecting acute rejection but lacks specificity. Percutaneous biopsy is safe and may be needed to establish the diagnosis.

22.2.3.3. Bladder Leak

Bladder and duodenal segment leaks can be seen in 10–20% of bladder-drained pancreas transplants. Ultrasound, CT scan, and MRI can identify abdominal fluid collections that could result from leaks. Ultrasound is limited by overlying abdominal gas. Conventional or scintigraphic cystograms can confirm the diagnosis.

22.2.3.4. Perigraft Collections

Pancreatic pseudocysts, abscesses, hematomas, and urinomas can develop posttransplant. Ultrasound, CT scan, and MRI can identify the collections. Percutaneous drainage may be necessary. Guidance for drainage is most easily performed with ultrasound or CT scan.

Chapter 23

Endoscopy in Liver Transplantation

Arthur J. Geller

23.1. UPPER AND LOWER GASTROINTESTINAL ENDOSCOPY

In general, cancer must be ruled out in all patients awaiting organ transplantation. The endoscopist plays a definite role in this, especially in patients with end-stage liver disease. *Upper gastrointestinal endoscopy* is indicated in the preoperative evaluation of patients awaiting orthotopic liver transplantation. The rationale for performing this procedure in patients with advanced liver disease is to demonstrate the presence of lesions associated with portal hypertension, such as large esophageal varices, which may affect survival and may be treated with beta-blockers or band ligation.

The rationale for performing preoperative *colonoscopy* is to diagnose and to treat neoplastic lesions. If a cancer were diagnosed, curative resection, if possible, would be required prior to consideration of performing transplantation. Conversely, metastatic cancer is a contraindication to liver transplantation. Neither the underlying cause of the liver disease nor the Child–Pugh–Turcotte score apparently impacts the likelihood of finding a colon lesion. Thus, screening is carried out as it would be done in the general population, and patients older than 50 years should undergo screening examination of the colon. Preoperative colonoscopy should be performed in patients with primary sclerosing cholangitis and associated inflammatory bowel disease because of the increased risk of colonic dysplasia and cancer.

There are potentially *increased risks* in performing endoscopic procedures on patients who have advanced liver disease. Excessive bleeding may occur secondary to coagulopathy and to thrombocytopenia. Altered metabolism of sedative/hypnotic medication may lead to oversedation and/or overt encephalopathy. Postcolonoscopy peritonitis in patients with ascites is another potential complication.

23.2. ROLE OF ENDOSCOPIC RETROGRADE CHOLANGIOGRAPHY (ERCP) IN LIVER TRANSPLANTATION

23.2.1. Preoperative Evaluation and Treatment

The endoscopic management of symptomatic dominant strictures in patients with primary sclerosing cholangitis includes balloon dilation and/or placement of a biliary endoprosthesis (stent). These interventions are successful in the majority of patients and have been demonstrated to delay the need for liver transplantation. In patients who are candidates for liver transplantation, endoscopic therapy of dominant strictures is clearly preferable to surgical reconstruction, because biliary surgery makes the subsequent transplant procedure more technically difficult. Endoscopic techniques used to demonstrate the presence of cholangiocarcinoma before transplantation include brush cytology and biopsy performed through the ERCP scope. Unfortunately, while the specificity is excellent, the sensitivity of these procedures is poor. Occult cholangiocarcinoma is thus found in the resected hepatectomy specimen in approximately 10% of transplants performed for end-stage primary sclerosing cholangitis.

23.2.2. Postoperative Biliary Complications

Biliary complications may occur in up to one-third of liver transplant recipients. In the majority of adults undergoing liver transplantation, a choledocho-choledochostomy (CC) reconstruction is created in which there is a direct duct-to-duct anastomosis with or without a T tube. Conversely, in the vast majority of children, in all patients with primary sclerosing cholangitis, as well as a majority of those patients who require repeat transplantation, a choledochojejunostomy as Roux-en-Y (CJRY) is performed. The Roux limb varies typically between 20 and 40 cm of jejunum. This anatomy makes access to the anastomosis by ERCP difficult; therefore, a percutaneous transhepatic cholangiogram is usually required to evaluate biliary complications post-CJRY.

The risk of biliary complications posttransplant is increased in certain situations, including *hepatic artery thrombosis*, reduced-size grafts, prolonged allograft ischemia, and harvesting injuries. Hepatic artery thrombosis may occur in up to 10% of transplants in adults and a higher proportion in children. The donor common bile duct depends on the hepatic artery solely for its blood supply. Thus, bile duct ischemia is likely in the setting of hepatic artery thrombosis.

Reduced-size grafts are associated with a high frequency of biliary strictures. Possible causes for this association are prolonged ischemic time and chronic rejection. In itself, prolonged cold-ischemic time is associated with biliary complications such as stricture formation, epithelial sloughing, and biliary cast and sludge formation. The dissection performed during graft harvesting may compromise the blood supply to the proximal biliary tree of the donor liver in the absence of proximal hepatic artery obstruction. Portal vein thrombosis is also associated with a high frequency of biliary complications.

A donor *cystic duct mucocele* may develop as a result of continued mucous production in a segment of cystic duct ligated proximally and distally at a distance. The enlarging mass may cause a biliary obstruction in a manner analogous to Mirizzi's syndrome. The lesion may be demonstrated by ERCP but is not amenable to endoscopic therapy and requires surgery.

23.2.3. Management of Biliary Complications

23.2.3.1. Bile Leaks

Bile leaks (Fig. 23.1) are the most common type of biliary complication following liver transplantation. Multiple factors are believed to be responsible for the development of leaks in the early postoperative period. These early leaks are diagnosed in the initial hospitalization and typically occur at the anastomosis of a CC. The cause is related to poor healing, ischemia, and technical factors, such as tension on the anastomosis. Leakage at the T-tube insertion site may also occur early in the postoperative course. Other, less common causes are leaks related to the cut surface of a reduced-size graft, cystic duct leaks, and damage to accessory ducts. Leaks associated with the T tube typically occur approximately 4 months posttransplantation. The T tube is placed approximately 1 cm distal to the CC anastomosis on the contralateral side of the hepatic artery anastomosis. The routine use of T tubes has recently been called into question. Corticosteroids, used in the immunosuppressive protocol, are believed to play a role by inhibiting the formation of a mature fibrous tract, thus promoting the development of a leak.

Various endoscopic (ERCP) techniques have been employed in the management of bile leaks: *sphincterotomy, nasobiliary tube placement,* and *endoprosthesis (stent) placement.* In all of these therapies, the sphincter of Oddi pressure gradient is eliminated, equalizing the pressure in the common bile duct with that in the duodenum, and allowing bile to flow into the duodenum and away from the leak, permitting closure.

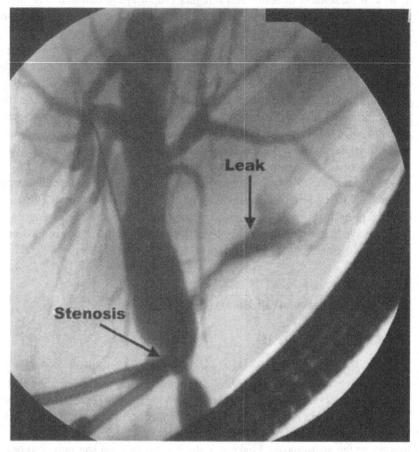

Figure 23.1. ERCP image of a biliary leak with an associated anastomotic stenotic area.

Nasobiliary tube or stent placement without sphincterotomy is preferable because of the increased risks associated with sphincterotomy, such as bleeding, pancreatitis, and perforation. The advantage of the nasobiliary tube over the stent is the ability to perform interval cholangiograms easily and to remove the tube without a second endoscopic procedure. The majority of leaks (90%) can be successfully sealed with these techniques. The mean time to leak closure with the nasobiliary tube is approximately 5 days, with a range of 2–13 days. Stents have also been reported to treat leaks successfully after being left in place approximately 6–8 weeks.

23.2.3.2. Biliary Strictures

Postoperative biliary strictures (Fig. 23.2) may be classified as anastomotic or nonanastomotic. The pathogenesis of *anastomotic strictures* is related to technical factors as well as to local ischemia and fibrosis. Nonanastomotic strictures involve vascular and endothelial damage.

Hepatic artery thrombosis (HAT) is an important factor in the pathogenesis of strictures. Factors related to HAT include surgical technique, small vessel size, hypercoagulability, prolonged cold-ischemic time, and ABO blood group incompatibility. *Immunologic injury* may play a role in stricture formation. Patients with chronic ductopenic rejection and those transplanted with an ABO incompatible graft are at increased risk for the development of strictures. Patients who undergo transplantation because of *primary sclerosing cholangitis* are also at increased risk for the development of strictures.

Endoscopic management of biliary strictures is aimed at preventing complications of strictures such as choledocholithiasis, cholangitis, and biliary cirrhosis, while avoiding the need for surgery. Stricture dilation using balloon dilators is performed. Subsequently, stent placement is performed.

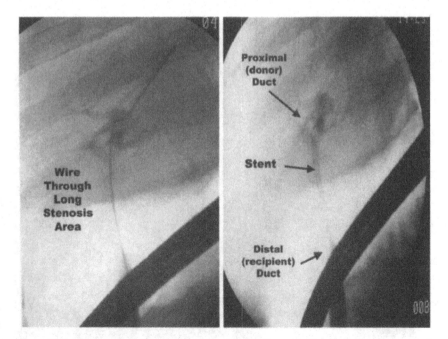

Figure 23.2. ERCP image of a long stenosis/stricture before and after successful placement of transanastomotic stent.

Nonanastomotic strictures (those involving the donor hepatic duct) are often associated with HAT, cholangitis, and choledocholithiasis, and are often multiple. These strictures are more difficult to treat and require more prolonged stenting. Rizk et al. (*Gastrointest Endosc* 1998;*47*:128–135), utilizing repeat ERCP and stent changes at 8- to 12-week intervals to prevent the complication of cholangitis secondary to stent occlusion, found that 22 months after the first ERCP procedure, 73% of patients with donor hepatic duct stricture were stent-free compared to 90% of patients with anastomotic stricture.

23.2.3.3.   Bile Duct Dilatation

A mild increase of 1–2 mm in the caliber of the extrahepatic ducts has been reported posttransplantation. Biliary (Fig. 23.3) enlargement may be a benign finding or may indicate a pathological process. Sossenheimer et al. (*Endoscopy* 1996;*28*:565–571) have pointed out that although diffuse dilation of the bile duct is thought to be due to denervation of the native duct, normal sphincter of Oddi function has been demonstrated posttransplantation. Findings suggestive of obstruction are a larger duct caliber (> 12 mm), cystic duct remnant dilatation, and

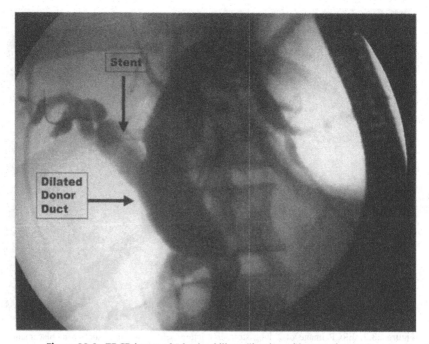

Figure 23.3. ERCP image of a benign biliary dilatation with stent placement.

abnormal liver enzymes. In this setting, a mechanical obstruction such as choledocholithiasis or sphincter of Oddi dysfunction (SOD) should be considered.

Liver enzyme improvement, with unclamping of the T tube, delayed contrast drainage on cholangiography, and delayed biliary drainage on hepatobiliary scintigraphy, supports the presence of an obstructive process. Performance of ERCP will rule out distal obstruction caused by stones, or distal strictures and sphincter of Oddi manometry may demonstrate SOD. Depending on the center and the allograft function, observation, endoscopic sphincterotomy, or CJRY may be performed for diffuse dilation of donor and recipient duct.

23.2.3.4. Choledocholithiasis and Biliary Sludge

Biliary calculi may be pigmented or cholesteric in nature. Predisposing factors are biliary obstruction, infection, and epithelial sloughing. Biliary sludge may be composed of unconjugated bilirubin or of casts of the duct comprising connective tissue and the lining wall of the bile duct. These are more common in cases of long-standing biliary obstruction or stenosis, HAT, prolonged cold preservation times (> 12 h), ABO-incompatible liver donors, or non-heart-beating liver donors. Endoscopic evaluation and treatment include ERCP to identify the debris and to assess for a predisposing obstructive lesion, such as a stricture. Endoscopic sphincterotomy and duct clearance are also performed at the time of ERCP to remove the debris. Alternatively, in the absence of HAT, CJRY reconstruction may be performed.

Suggested Reading

REFERENCE TEXTBOOKS

Auchincloss H, Shaffer D. Pancreas transplantation. In: Ginns LC, Cosimi AB, Morris PJ, Eds., *Transplantation* (pp. 395–421). Malden, MA: Blackwell Science, 1999.

Bussutil RW, Klintmalm GB, eds. *Transplantation of the Liver*. Philadelphia: W. B. Saunders, 1996.

Cecka JM, Terasaki PI, eds. *Clinical Transplants 1999*. Los Angeles, UCLA Tissue Typing Laboratory, 1999.

Child CG, Turcotte JG. *Surgery and Portal Hypertension: The Liver and Portal Hypertension*. Philadelphia: W. B. Saunders, 1964.

Flye MW, ed. *Principles of Organ Transplantation*. Philadelphia: W. B. Saunders, 1989.

Greenberg A, ed. *Primary on Kidney Diseases* (2nd ed.). San Diego. CA: Academic Press, 1997.

Jennette JC, Schwartz ML, Silva FG, eds. *Hepinstall's Pathology of the Kidney*. Philadelphia: Lippincott–Raven, 1998.

Kandarpa K, Gardiner GA. Angiography. In: Kandarpa K, Aruny JE, Eds., *Handbook of Interventional Radiologic Procedures* (pp. 3–26). Boston: Little, Brown, 1996.

Malloy PC, Marx MV. Diagnosis and management of biliary complications after orthotopic liver transplantation. In: LaBerge Jm, Venbrux AC, Eds., *Biliary Interventions* (pp. 259–280). San Francisco: Society of Cardiovascular and Interventional Radiology, 1995.

Morris PJ, ed. *Kidney Transplantation: Principles and Practice* (4th ed.). Philadelphia: W. B. Saunders, 1994.

Norman DJ, Suki WN, eds. *Primer on Transplantation*. Thorofare, NJ: American Society of Transplant Physicians, 1998.

Pathology of renal transplantation. In: Kern WF, Classic ZG, Nadasy T, Silva FG, Bane BL, Pitha JV, Eds., *Atlas of Renal Pathology* (pp. 247–260). Philadelphia: W. B. Saunders, 1999.

Sale GE, Snover DC, Radio SJ. Transplantation pathology. In: Damjanov J, Linder F, Eds., *Anderson's Pathology* (10th ed.). St. Louis, MO: Mosby, 1996.

Trzepacz PT, DiMartini A, eds. *The Transplant Patient: Biological, Psychiatric and Ethical Issued in Organ Transplantation*. Cambridge, UK: Cambridge University Press, 2000.

ARTICLES

Pretransplant Evaluation, Selection, and Management

Achord JL. Malnutrition and the role of nutritional support in alcoholic liver disease. *Am J Gastroenterol* 1987;*82*:1–7.

Andreu M, Sola R, Sitges-Serra A, et al. Risk factors for spontaneous bacterial peritonitis in cirrhotic patients with ascites. *Gastroenterology* 1993;*104*:1133–1138.

Arroyo V, Gines P, Gerbes AL, Dudley FJ, Gentilini P, Laffi G, Reynolds TB, Ring-Larsen H, Scholmerich J. Definition and diagnostic criteria of refractory ascites and hepatorenal syndrome in cirrhosis: International Ascites Club. *Hepatology* 1996;*23*:164–176.

Badalamenti S, Graziani G, Salerno F, Ponticelli C. Hepatorenal syndrome: New perspectives in pathogenesis and treatment. *Arch Intern Med* 1993;*153*:1957–1967.

Bernard B, Lebrec D, Mathurin P, Opolon P, Poynard T. Propranolol and sclerotherapy in the prevention of gastrointestinal rebleeding in patients with cirrhosis: A meta-analysis. *J Hepatol* 1997;*26*:312–324.

Boker KH, Dalley G, Bahr MJ, et al. Long-term outcome of hepatitis C virus infection after liver transplantation. *Hepatology* 1997;*25*:203–210.

Cooper GS, Bellamy P, Dawson NV, et al. A prognostic model for patients with end-stage liver disease. *Gastroenterology* 1997;*113*(4):1278–1288.

Corry RJ, Zehr P. Quality of life in diabetic recipients of kidney transplants is better with the addition of the pancreas. *Clin Transpl* 1990;*4*(4):238–241.

D'Amico G, Morabito A, Pagliaro L, Marubini E. Survival and prognostic indicators in compensated and decompensated cirrhosis. *Dig Dis Sci* 1986; *31*:468–475.

D'Amico G, Pagliaro L, Bosch J. The treatment of portal hypertension: A meta-analytic review. *Hepatology* 1995;*22*:332–354.

Dodson SF, Issa S, Bonham A. Liver transplantation for chronic viral hepatitis. *Surg Clin North Am* 1999;*79*(1):131–145.

Eggers PW. Effect of transplantation on the Medicare End-Stage Renal Disease Program. *N Engl J Med* 1988;*318*:223–239.

Farmer DG, Rosove MH, Shaked A, Busuttil RW. Current treatment modalities for hepatocellular carcinoma. *Ann Surg* 1994;*219*:236–247.

Farney AC, Cho E, Schweitzer EJ, et al. Simultaneous cadaver pancreas living donor kidney transplantation: A new approach for the type 1 diabetic uremic patient. *Ann Surg* 2000;*232*(5):696–703.

Ferenci P, Herneth A, Steindl P. Newer approaches to therapy of hepatic encephalopathy. *Semin Liver Dis* 1996;*16*:329–338.

Fingerote RJ, Bain VG. Fulminant hepatic failure. *Am J Gastroenterol* 1995;*88*(7):1000.

Fong TL, Akriviadis EA, Runyon BA, Reynolds TB. Polymorphonuclear cell count response and duration of antibiotic therapy in spontaneous bacterial peritonitis. *Hepatology* 1989;*9*:423–426.

Greenstein S, Siegal B. Evaluation of a multivariate model predicting noncompliance with medication regimens among renal transplant patients. *Transplantation* 2000;*69*(10):2226–2228.

Halpern EJ, Mitchell DJ, Wechsler RJ, Outwater EK, Mortiz MJ, Wilson GA. Preoperative evaluation of living renal donors: Comparison of CT angiography and MR angiography. *Radiology* 2000;*216*(2):434–439.

Hillaire S, Labianca M, Borgonovo G, Smadja C, Grange D, Franco D. Peritoneovenous shunting of intractable ascites in patients with cirrhosis: Improving results and predictive factors of failure. *Surgery* 1993;*113*:373–379.

Hobnailed JH, Kresina T, Fuller RK, et al. Liver transplantation for alcoholic liver disease: Executive statement and recommendations. Summary of a National Institutes of Health workshop held December 6–7, 1996, Bethesda, MD. *Liver Transpl Surg* 1997;*3*(3), 347–350.

Hughes RD, Williams R. Evaluation of extracorporeal bioartificial liver devices. *Liver Transpl Surg* 1995;*1*:200.

Humar A, Sutherland DER, Ramcharan T, et al. Optimal timing for a pancreas transplant after a successful kidney transplant. *Transplantation* 2000;*70*(8):1247–1250.

Inadomi J, Sonnenberg A. Cost-analysis of prophylactic antibiotics in spontaneous bacterial peritonitis. *Gastroenterology* 1997;*113*:1289–1294.

International Pancreas Transplant Registry Annual Report for 1998, Vol. 11(1), May 1999.

Jurim O, Shakleton CR, McDiarmid SV, et al. Living donor liver transplantation at UCLA. *Am J Surg* 1995;*169*:529–532.

Keefe EB. Summary of guidelines on organ allocation and patient listing for liver transplantation. *Liver Transpl Surg* 1998;*4*(Suppl 1):S108–S114.

Kim WR, Wiesner RH, Therneau TM, et al. Optimal timing of liver transplantation for primary biliary cirrhosis. *Hepatology* 1998;*28*(1):33–38.

Kleber G, Sauerbruch T, Ansari H, Paumgartner G. Prediction of variceal hemorrhage in cirrhosis: A prospective follow-up study. *Gastroenterology* 1991;*100*:1332–1337.

Kondrup J, Muller MJ. Energy and protein requirements of patients with chronic liver disease. *J Hepatol* 1997;*27*:239–247.

Krowka MJ. Hepatopulmonary syndrome: What are we learning from interventional radiology, liver transplantation, and other disorders? *Gastroenterology* 1995;*109*:1009–1013.

Kuo PC, Johnson LB, Schweitzer EJ, et al. Solitary pancreas allografts: The role of percutaneous biopsy and standardized histologic grading of rejection. *Arch Surg* 1997;*132*:52–57.

Lake JR. Changing indications for liver transplantation. *Gastroenterol Clin North Am* 1993;*22*(2): 213–329.

Levenson JL, Olbrisch ME. Psychosocial evaluation of organ transplant candidates: A comparative survey of process, criteria and outcomes in heart, liver, and kidney transplant programs. *Psychosomatics* 1993;*34*:314–323.

Lewis DA, Smith RE: Steroid-induced psychiatric syndromes. *J Affect Disord* 1983;*5*:319–332.

Lidofsky SD, Bass NM, Prager MC, et al. Intracranial pressure monitoring and liver transplantation for fulminant hepatic failure. *Hepatology* 1992;*16*:1–7.

Linas SL, Schaefer JW, Moore EE, Good JT, Jr, Giansiracusa R. Peritoneovenous shunt in the management of the hepatorenal syndrome. *Kidney Int* 1986;*30*:736–740.

Lucey MR, Brown KA, Everson GT, et al. Minimal criteria for placement of adults on the liver transplant waiting list: A report of a national conference organized by the American Society of Transplant Physicians and the American Association for the Study of Liver Diseases. *Liver Transpl Surg* 1997;*3*(6):628–637.

Luxon BA. Liver transplantation: Who should be referred—and when? *Postgrad Med* 1997; *102*(6):103–113.

Markman JF, Markowitz JS, Yersiz H, et al. Long term survival after retransplantation of the liver. *Ann Surg* 1997;*26*(4):418–420.

Matsuzaki Y, Tanaka N, Osuga T, et al. Improvement of biliary enzyme levels and itching as a result of long-term administration of ursodeoxycholic acid in primary biliary cirrhosis. *Am J Gastroenterol* 1990;*85*:15–23.

Mazzaferro V, Regalia E, Doci R, et al. Liver transplantation for the treatment of hepatocellular carcinomas in patients with cirrhosis. *N Engl J Med* 1996;*334*:693–699.

McCune TR, Nylander WA, Van Buren DH, et al. Colonic screening prior to renal transplantation and its impact on post-transplant colonic complications. *Clin Transpl* 1992;*6*(2):91–96.

McGory RW, Ishitani MB, Oliveira WM, et al. Improved outcome of orthotopic liver transplantation for chronic hepatitis B cirrhosis with aggressive–passive immunization. *Liver Transplantation* 1992;*61*:1358–1364.

Mori DA, Klein W, Gallager P. Validity of the MMPI-2 and Beck Depression Inventory for making decisions of organ allocation in renal transplantation. *Psychological Reports* 1999;*84*:114–116.

National Institutes of Health Consensus. Development Conference Statement: Liver Transplantation, June 20–23, 1983. *Hepatology* 1984;*4*:107–110. Bethesda, MD: National Institutes of Health.

O'Grady JR, Alexander GJM, Hayllar KM, et al. Early indicators of prognosis in fulminant hepatic failure. *Gastroenterology* 1989;*97*:439–445.

Olbrisch ME, Levenson JL. Psychosocial assessment of organ transplant candidates: Current status of methodological and philosophical issues. *Psychosomatics* 1995;*36*:236–243.

Pagliaro L, D'Amico G, Sorensen TI, et al. Prevention of first bleeding in cirrhosis. A meta-analysis of randomized trials of nonsurgical treatment. *Ann Intern Med* 1992;*117*:59–70.

Pauwels A, Mostefa-Kara N, Debenes B, Degoutte E, Levy VG. Systemic antibiotic prophylaxis after gastrointestinal hemorrhage in cirrhotic patients with a high risk of infection. *Hepatology* 1996;*24*:802–806.

Penn I. The effect of immunosuppression on pre-existing cancers. *Liver Transplantation* 1993;*55*: 742–747.

Penn I. Evaluation of transplant candidates with pre-existing malignancies. *Ann Transpl Surg* 1997;*2*(4):14–17.

Perrillo R, Rakela J, Martin P, et al. Long-term lamivudine therapy of patients with recurrent hepatitis B post liver transplantation. *Hepatology* 1997;*26*:177A.

Ploeg RJ, D'Alessandro AM, Knechtle SJ, et al. Risk factors for primary dysfunction after liver transplantation—a multivariate analysis. *Transplantation* 1993;*55*(4):807–813.

Podesta A, Lopez P, Terg R, et al. Treatment of pruritus of primary biliary cirrhosis with rifampin. *Dig Dis Sci* 1991;*36*:216–220.

Rebibou JM, Chabod J, Bittencourt MC, et al. Flow-PRA evaluation for antibody screening in patients awaiting kidney transplantation. *Transpl Immunol* 2000;*8*(2):125–128.

Rosen HR, Shackleton CR, Martin P. Indications for and timing of liver transplantation. *Med Clin North Am* 1996;*80*(5):1069–1102.

Runyon BA. Management of adult patients with ascites caused by cirrhosis. *Hepatology* 1998;*27*:264–272.

Runyon BA, Antillon MR, Akriviadis EA, McHutchison JG. Bedside inoculation of blood culture bottles with ascitic fluid is superior to delayed inoculation in the detection of spontaneous bacterial peritonitis. *J Clin Microbiol* 1990;*28*:2811–2812.

Runyon BA, McHutchison JG, Antillon MR, Akriviadis EA, Montano AA. Short-course versus long-course antibiotic treatment of spontaneous bacterial peritonitis: A randomized controlled study of 100 patients [see comments]. *Gastroenterology* 1991;*100*:1737–1742.

Ryes J. Iwatsuki S. Current management of portal hypertension with liver transplantation. *Adv Surg* 1992;*25*:189.

Saab S, Han S, Martin P. Liver transplantation: Selection, listing criteria, and preoperative management. *Clinics in Liver Disease* 2000:*4*(3):513–532.

Sanyal AJ. The management of the cirrhotic patient after transjugular intrahepatic portosystemic shunt. *Semin Gastrointest Dis* 1997;*8*:188–199.

Sanyal AJ, Freedman Am, Luketic VA, et al. Transjugular intrahepatic portosystemic shunts compared with endoscopic sclerotherapy for the prevention of recurrent variceal hemorrhage: A randomized, controlled trial. *Ann Intern Med* 1997;*126*:849–857.

Sarin SK, Lamba GS, Kumar M, Misra A, Murthy NS. Comparison of endoscopic ligation and propranolol for the primary prevention of variceal bleeding [see comments]. *N Engl J Med* 1999;*340*:988–993.

Schalm SW, van Buren HR. Prevention of recurrent variceal bleeding: Non-surgical procedures. *Clin Gastroenterol* 1985; *14*:209–232.

Schneider AW, Kalk JF, Klein CP. Effect of losartan, an angiotensin II receptor antagonist, on portal pressure in cirrhosis. *Hepatology* 1999;*29*:334–339.

Sheiner PA, Schluger LK, Emre S, et al. Retransplantation for recurrent hepatitis C. *Liver Transpl Surg* 1997;*3*:130–136.

Shiffman ML, Jeffers L, Hoofnagle JH, Tralka TS. The role of transjugular intrahepatic portosystemic shunt for treatment of portal hypertension and its complications: A conference sponsored by the National Digestive Diseases Advisory Board. *Hepatology* 1995;*22*:1591–1597.

Somberg KA, Lake JR, Doherty MM, et al. The clinical course following transjugular intrahepatic portosystemic shunts (TIPS) in liver transplant candidates. *Hepatology* 1993;*18*:103A.

Stanley MM, Ochi S, Lee KK, Nemchausky BA, Greenlee HB, Allen JI, Allen MJ, Baum RA, Gadacz TR, Camara DS. Peritoneovenous shunting as compared with medical treatment in patients with alcoholic cirrhosis and massive ascites. Veterans Administration Cooperative Study on Treatment of Alcoholic Cirrhosis with Ascites. *N Engl J Med* 1989;*321*:1632–1638.

Steiber AC, Gordon RD, Todo S. et al. Liver transplantation in patients over sixty years of age. *Liver Transplantation* 1991;*51*:271–273.

Stratta RJ, Taylor RJ, Lowell JA, et al. Preemptive combined pancreas kidney transplantation: Is earlier better? *Trans Proc* 1994;*26*(2):422–424.

Teran JC, Imperiale TF, Mullen KD, Tavill AS, McCullough AJ. Primary prophylaxis of variceal bleeding in cirrhosis: A cost-effectiveness analysis. *Gastroenterology* 1997;*112*:473–482.

Terra SG, Tsunoda SM. Opioid antagonists in the treatment of pruritus from cholestatic liver disease. *Ann Pharmacother* 1998;*32*:1228–1230.

Tito L, Rimola A, Gines P, Llach J, Arroyo V, Rodes J. Recurrence of spontaneous bacterial peritonitis in cirrhosis: Frequency and predictive factors. *Hepatology* 1988;8:27–31.

Trevitt R, Whittaker C, Ball EA. Evaluation of potential transplant recipients and living donors [Review]. *EDTNA ERCA J* 2000;*26*(1):26–28.

Tzakis AG, Cooper MH, Dummer JS, et al. Liver transplantation in HIV + patients. *Liver Transplantation* 1990;*49*:354–358.

Uriz J, Gines P, Cardenas A. et al. Terlipressin plus albumin infusion: An effective and safe therapy of hepatorenal syndrome. *J Hepatol* 2000;*33*:43–48.

Weisner RH. Liver transplantation for primary biliary cirrhosis and primary sclerosing cholangitis: Predicting outcomes with natural history models. *Mayo Clin Proc* 1998;*73*:575–588.

Wong T, Devlin J, Rolando N, Heaton N. Williams R. Clinical characteristics affecting the outcome of liver retransplantation. *Transplantation* 1997;*64*(6):878–882.

Organ Donation, Procurement, and Allocation

Broelsch CE, Burdelski M, Rogiers X, et al. Living-donor for liver transplantation. *Hepatology* 1994;*20*:49S–55S.

Caplan A. Must I be my brother's keeper? Ethical issues in the use of living donors as sources of liver and other solid organs. *Transpl Proc* 1993;*25*:1997–2000.

Darby JM, Stein K, Grenvik A, Stuart SA. Approach to management of the heartbeating "brain dead" organ donor. *JAMA* 1989;*261*:2222–2228.

Johnson EM, Remucal MJ, Gillingham KJ, et al. Complications and risks of living donor nephrectomy. *Transplantation* 1997;*64*:1124–1128.

Kasiske BL, Bia MJ. The evaluation and selection of living kidney donors. *Am J Kidney Dis* 1995;*26*:387–398.

Marcos A. Right lobe living donor liver transplantation. *Transplantation* 1999;*68*(6):798–803.

Matas AJ, Najarian JS. Kidney transplantation—the living donor. In: Terasaki PI, Cecka JM, eds. *Clinical Transplants 1994.* Los Angeles: Immunogenetics Center, 1995.

Miller CM, Mazzaferro V, Makowka L, et al. Rapid flush technique for donor hepatectomy: Safety and efficacy of an improved method of liver recovery for transplantation. *Transpl Proc* 1988;*20*: 948–950.

Ratner LE, Kavoussi LR, Sroka M, et al. Laparoscopic assisted live donor nephrectomy—a comparison with the open approach. *Transplantation* 1997;*63*:229–233.

Soifer BE, Gelf AW. The multiple organ donor: Identification and management. *Ann Intern Med* 1989;*110*:814–823.

Starzl TE, Miller CM, Rappaport FT. Algorithm and explanation: Approach to the potential organ donor. American College of Surgeons. Care of the surgical patient, elective care. Chapter XI: Miscellaneous care problems. *Scientific American* 1990.

Tan HP, Kavoussi LR, Sosa JA, Montgomery RA, Ratner LE. Laparoscopic live donor nephrectomy: Debating the benefits. *Nephrology News and Issues* 1999;*11*:90–95.

Tanaka K, Uemoto S, Tkunaga Y, et al. Surgical techniques and innovations in living-related liver transplantation. *Ann Surg* 1993;*217*:82–91.

Terasaki PI, Cecka JM, Gjertson DW, et al. High survival rates of kidney transplants from spousal and living unrelated donors. *N Engl J Med* 1995;*333*:333–336.

Todo S, Makowka L, Tzakis AG, et al. Hepatic artery in liver transplantation. *Transpl Proc* 1987;*19*:2406–2411.

Operative and Postoperative Care and Complications

Afessa B, Gay PC, Plevak DJ, et al. Pulmonary complications or orthotopic liver transplantation. *Mayo Clin Proc* 1993;*68*:427–434.

Basadonna GP, Matas AJ, Gillinghan KJ, et al. Early versus late acute renal allograft rejection: Impact on chronic rejection. *Transplantation* 1993;*55*:993–995.

Bronster DJ, Emre S, et al. Neurological complications of orthotopic liver transplantation. *Mt Sinai J Med* 1994;*61*:63–69.

Canzanello VJ, Schwartz L, Taler SJ, Textor SC, Wiesner RH, Porayko MK, et al. Evolution of cardiovascular risk after liver transplantation: A comparison of cyclosporine A and tacrolimus (FK506). *Liver Transpl Surg* 1997;*3*:1–9.

Ciancio G, Julian JF, Fernandez L, Miller J, Burke GW. Successful surgical salvage of pancreas allografts after complete venous thrombosis. *Transplantation* 2000;*70*(1):126–131.

Ciancio G, Olson L, Burke GW. The use of the brachiocephalic trunk for arterial reconstruction of the whole pancreas allograft for transplantation. *J Am Coll Surg* 1995;*181*:79.

D'Alessandro AM, Ploeg RJ, Knechtle SJ, et al. Retransplantation of the liver–a seven year experience. *Transplantation* 1993;*55*:1083–1087.

Dodd GD, Memel DS, Zajko AB, et al. Hepatic artery stenosis and thrombosis in transplant recipients: Doppler diagnosis with resistive index and systolic acceleration time. *Radiology* 1994;*192*: 657–661.

Dominguez J, Clase CM, Mahalti K, et al. Is routine ureteric stenting needed in kidney transplantation? A randomized trial. *Transplantation* 2000;*70*(4):597–601.

Emond JC, Whittington PF, Thistlethwaite JR, et al. Transplantation of two patients with one liver. *Ann Surg* 1990;*212*:14–22.

Galazka Z, Szmidt J, Nazarewski S, et al. Kidney transplantation in recipients with atherosclerotic iliac vessels. *Ann Transpl* 1999;*4*(2):43–44.

Gill IS, Sindhi R, Jerius JT, Sudan D, Stratta RJ. Bench reconstruction of pancreas for transplantation: Experience with 192 cases. *Clin Transplants* 1997;*2*:104–109.

Goldstein RM, Secrest CL, Klintmalm GB, et al. Problematic vascular reconstruction in liver transplantation: Part I. Arterial. *Surgery* 1990;*107*:540–543.

Greig PD, Woolf GM, Abecassis M, et al. Treatment of primary liver graft nonfunction with prostaglandin E. *Transplantation* 1989;*48*:447–453.

Gruessner AC, Sutherland DER. Pancreas transplants for United States and non US cases as reported to the International Pancreas Transplant Registry (IPTR) and to the United Network for Organ Sharing (UNOS). In: Cecka JM, Terasacki PI, eds. *Clinical Transplants 1997*. Los Angeles: UCLA Tissue Typing Laboratory, 1998.

Humar A, Kandaswamy R, et al. Decreased surgical risks of pancreas transplantation in the modern era. *Ann Surg* 2000;*231*(2):269–275.

Jurim O, Shaked A, Kiai K, et al. Celiac compression syndrome and liver transplantation. *Ann Surg* 1993;*218*(1):10–12.

Kahl A, Bechstein WO, Frei U. Trends and perspectives in pancreas and simultaneous pancreas and kidney transplantation. *Curr Opin Urol* 2001;*11*(2):165–174.

Kirsch JP, Howard TK, Klintmalm GB, et al. Problematic vascular reconstruction in liver transplantation: Part II. Portovenous conduits. *Surgery* 1990;*107*:544–548.

Langnas AN, Marujo W, Stratta RJ, Wood RP, Shaw BW. Vascular complications after orthotopic liver transplantation. *Am J Surg* 1991;*161*:76.

Lerut J, Tzakis AG, Bron KM, et al. Complications of venous reconstruction in human orthotopic liver transplantation. *Ann Surg* 1986;*205*:404.

Matas AJ, Gillingham KJ, et al. Immunologic and nonimmunologic factors: Different risks for cadaver and living donor transplantation. *Transplantation* 2000;*69*:54–58.

Mazariegos GV, Molmenti EP, Kramer DJ. Early complications after liver transplantation. *Surg Clin North Am* 1999;*79*(1):109–129.

Mazzaferro V, Esquivel CO, Makowka L, et al. Hepatic artery thrombosis after pediatric liver transplantation—a medical or surgical event. *Transplantation* 1989;*47*:971–977.

Merkus JWS, Huysmans FTM, Hoitsma AJ, et al. Treatment of renal allograft artery stenosis. *Transpl Int* 1993;*6*:111.

O'Connor TP, Lewis WD, Jenkins RL. Biliary tract complications after liver transplantation. *Arch Surg* 1995;*130*:312–317.

Ostrowski M, Lubikowski J, Kowalczyk M, Power J. Laparoscopic lymphocele drainage after renal transplantation. *Ann Transpl* 2000;*5*(1):25–27.

Ostrowski M, Wlodarczyk Z, Wesolowski T, et al. Influence of ureterovesical anastomosis technique on the incidence of vesicoureteral reflux in renal transplant recipients. *Ann Transpl* 1999;*4*(1): 54–58.

Otte JB, DeVille De Goyet J, Sokal E, et al. Size reduction of the donor liver is a safe way to alleviate the shortage of size-matched organs in pediatric liver transplantation. *Ann Surg* 1990;*211*: 146–157.

Paul LC, Hayry P, Foegh M, et al. Diagnostic criteria for chronic rejection/accelerated graft atherosclerosis in heart and kidney transplants. *Transpl Proc* 1993;*25*:2022–2023.

Paya C. Controversies in transplant infection. *Transpl Proc* 1995;*27*(5, Suppl 1):23–24.

Paya CV, Herman PE, Wiesner RH, Ludwig J, Smith TF, Rakela J, et al. Cytomegalovirus hepatitis in liver transplantation: Prospective analysis of 93 consecutive orthotopic liver transplantations. *J Infect Dis* 1989;*160*:752–758.

Pleass HC, Clark KR, Rigg KM, et al. Urologic complications after renal transplantation: A prospective randomized trial comparing different techniques of ureteric anastomosis and the use of prophylactic ureteric stents. *Transpl Proc* 1995;*27*:1091.

Reyes J, Mazariegos GV. Pediatric transplantation [Review]. *Surg Clin North Am* 1999;*79*(1):163–189.

Schult M, Kuster J, Kliem V, et al. Native pyeloureterostomy after kidney transplantation: Experience in 48 cases. *Transpl Int* 2000;*13*(5):340–343.

Schurman SJ, McEnery PT. Factors influencing short term and long term pediatric renal transplant survival. *J Pediatr* 1997;*130*:455–462.

Shaked A, Busutil RW. Liver transplantation in patients with portal vein thrombosis and central porta caval shunts. *Ann Surg* 1991;*214*:696.

Shapira Z, Yussim A, Mor E. Pancreas transplantation [Review]. *J Pediatr Endocrinol Metab* 1999;*12*(1):3–15.

Singh N. The current management of infectious disease in the liver transplant recipient. *Clin Liver Dis* 2000;*4*(3):657–673.

Singh N, Gayowski T, Wagener M, et al. Pulmonary infiltrates in liver transplant recipients in the intensive care unit. *Transplantation* 1999;*67*:1138–1143.

Snowden CP, Hughes T, Rose J, et al. Pulmonary edema in patients after liver transplantation. *Liver Transplantation* 2000;*6*(4):466–470.

Stablein DM. After six thousand transplants where are we? The state of pediatric renal transplantation in North America. *Pediatr Transpl* 2000;*4*S105.

Stratta RJ, Gaber AO, Shokouh-Amiri MH, et al. Evolution in pancreas transplantation techniques: Simultaneous kidney–pancreas transplantation using portal-enteric drainage without anti-lymphocyte induction. *Ann Surg* 1999;*229*(5):701–708; discussion 709–712.

Stratta RJ, Wood RP, Langnas AN, et al. Diagnosis and treatment of biliary tract complications after orthotopic liver transplantation. *Clin Pharm Ther* 1989;*106*:675–684.

Takaoka F, Brown MR, Paulsen AW, et al. Adult respiratory distress syndrome following orthotopic liver transplantation. *Clin Transpl* 1989;*3*:294–299.

Troppmann C, Benedetti E, Gruessner AC, et al. Vascular graft thrombosis after pancreas transplantation: Uni and multivariate surgical and nonsurgical risk factor analysis. *J Am Coll Surg* 1996; *182*:285–316.

Troppmann C, Gruessner AC, Dunn DL, Sutherland DER, Gruessner RWG. Surgical complications requiring early relaparotomy after pancreas transplantation. *Ann Surg* 1998;*227*(2):255–268.

Tzakis A, Todo S, Stieber A, et al. Venous jump grafts for liver transplantation in patients with portal vein thrombosis. *Transplantation* 1989;*48*:530–531.

Winston DJ, Emmanoulides C, Busuttil RW. Infections in liver transplant recipients. *Clin Infect Dis* 1995;*21*:1077–1091.

Wright FH, Smith JL, Corry RJ. Postoperative complications of pancreas transplantation. *Diabetes* 1989;*39*:236–237.

Young JB. *Clinical Trends in Transplant Survival.* AST Lectures in Transplantation, November 2000.

Immunosuppression

Armenti VT, Moritz MJ, Radomski GA, et al. Pregnancy and transplantation. *Graft* 2000;*3*(2):59–62.

Burke GW, Ricordi C, Karatzas T, et al. Donor bone marrow infusion in simultaneous pancreas/kidney transplant recipients: A preliminary study. *Transpl Proc* 1995;*27*(6):3121–3122.

Cakaloglu Y, Tredger JM, Devlin J, Williams R. Importance of cytochrome P-450IIIA activity in determining dosage and blood levels of FK506 and cyclosporine in liver transplant recipients. *Hepatology* 1994;*20*:309–316.

Cosimi AB, Cho SI, Delmonico FL, Kaplan MM, Rohrer RJ, Jenkins RL. A randomized clinical trial comparing OKT3 and steroids for treatment of hepatic allograft rejection. *Transplantation* 1987;*43*:91–95.

Fraser GM, Grammoustianos K, Reddy J, Rolles K, Davidson B, Burroughs AK. Long-term immunosuppression without corticosteroids after orthotopic liver transplantation: A positive therapeutic aim. *Liver Transpl Surg* 1996;*2*:411–417.

Friese CE, Narumi S, Stock P, Melzer JS. Simultaneous pancreas–kidney transplantation: An overview of indications, complications and outcomes. *West J Med* 1999;*170*:11–18.

Fung JJ, Demetris AJ, Porter KA, et al. Use of OKT3 with cyclosporine and steroids for reversal of acute kidney and liver allograft rejection. *Nephron* 1987;*46*:19–33.

Fung JJ, Todo S, Jain A, et al. Conversion from cyclosporine to FK506 in liver allograft recipients with cyclosporine-related complications. *Transpl Proc* 1990;22:6–12.

Gruessner RW. Mycophenolate mofetil in pancreas transplantation. *Transplantation* 1998;66(3):318–323.

Hemming AW, Greig PD, Cattral MS, et al. A microemulsion of cyclosporine without intravenous cyclosporine in liver transplantation. *Transplantation* 1996;62:1798–1794.

Herrero JI, Quiroga J, Sangro B, et al. Conversation of liver transplant recipients on cyclosporine with renal impairment to mycophenolate mofetil. *Liver Transpl Surg* 1999;5:414–420.

International Pancreas Transplant Registry. Vol. 11(1), May 31, 1999.

Jordan ML. Results of pancreas transplantation after steroid withdrawal under tacrolimus immunosuppression. *Transplantation* 2000;69(2):265–271.

Klintmalm GB, Gonwa TA. Nephrotoxicity associated with cyclosporine and FK506. *Liver Transpl Surg* 1995;1:11–19.

McDiarmid S, Colonna J, Shaked A, Ament M, Busuttil R. A comparison of renal function in cyclosporine and FK506-treated patients after primary orthotopic liver transplantation. *Transplantation* 1993;56:847–853.

McMillan MA, Briggs JD, Junor BJ. Outcome of renal replacement therapy in patients with diabetes mellitus. *Br Med J* 1990;301:540–544.

Sollinger HW, Odorico JS, Knechtle SJ, et al. Experience with 500 simultaneous pancreas–kidney transplants. *Ann Surg* 1998;228:284–296.

Starzl TE, Hakala TR, Rosenthal JT, Iwatsuki S, Shaw BW. Variable convalescence and therapy after cadaveric renal transplantation under cyclosporine A and steroids. *Surg Gynecol Obstet* 1982;154:819–825.

Takaya S, Iwaki Y, Starzl TE. Liver transplantation in positive cytotoxic crossmatch cases using FK506, high-dose steroids, and prostaglandin El. *Transplantation* 1992;54:927–929.

Taler SJ, Textor SC, Canzanello VJ, et al. Role of steroid dose in hypertension early after liver transplantation with tacrolimus (FK506) and cyclosporine. *Transplantation* 1996;62:1588–1592.

Tesi RJ, Elkhammas EA, Henry ML, et al. Pattern of graft loss after combined kidney–pancreas transplant. *Transpl Proc* 1994;26(2):425–426.

Tran M, Larsen JL, Duckworth WC, et al. Anti-insulin antibodies are a cause of hypoglycemia following pancreas transplantation. *Diabetes Care* 1994;17:988–993.

Tyden G, Bolinder J, Solders G, et al. Improved survival in patients with insulin-dependent diabetes mellitus and end-stage diabetic nephropathy 10 years after combined pancreas and kidney transplantation. *Transplantation* 1999;67(5):645–648.

Diagnostic and Therapeutic Tools

Aideyan OA, Schmidt AJ, Trenkner SW, Hakim NS, Gruessner RW, Walsh JW. CT-guided percutaneous biopsy of pancreas transplants. *Radiology*, 1996; 201:825–828.

Bhagat VJ, Gordon RL, Osorio RW, et al. Ureteral obstruction and leaks after renal transplantation: Outcome of percutaneous antegrade ureteral stent placement in patients. *Radiology* 1998; 209:159–167.

Bourgeois N, Deviere J, Yeaton P, Bourgeois F, Adler M, Van De Stadt J, Gelin M, Cremer M. Diagnostic and therapeutic endoscopic retrograde cholangiography after liver transplantation. *Gastrointest Endosc* 1995;42:527–534.

Brown ED, Chen MYM, Wolfman NT, Ott DJ, Watson NE. Complications of renal transplantation: Evaluation with US and radionuclide imaging. *RadioGraphics* 2000;20:607–622.

Caridi JG, Devane AM, Hawkins IF, Newman R. Examination of renal donors using intraarterial digital subtraction angiography and a pigtail catheter. *Am J Radiol* 1997;169:537–539.

Dravid VS, Shapiro MJ, Needleman L, et al. Arterial abnormalities following orthotopic liver transplantation: Arteriographic findings and correlation with doppler sonographic findings. *Am J Radiol* 1994;*163*:585–589.

Dubovsky EV, Russell CD, Erbas B. Radionuclide evaluation of renal transplants. *Semin Nucl Med* 1995;25:49–59.

Freese DK, Snover DC, Sharp HI, et al. Chronic rejection after liver transplantation: A study of clinical, histopathological and immunological features. *Hepatology* 1991;*13*:882–891.

Krebs TL, Daly B, Wong JJ, Chow CC, Bartlett ST. Vascular complications of pancreatic transplantation: MR evaluation. *Radiology* 1995;*196*:793–798.

Krebs TL, Daly B, Wong-You-Cheong JJ, Carroll K, Bartlett ST. Acute pancreatic transplant rejection: Evaluation with dynamic contrast-enhanced MR imaging compared with histopathologic analysis. *Radiology* 1999;*210*:437–342.

Laghi A, Pavone P, Catalano C, et al. MR cholangiography of late biliary complications after liver transplantation. *Am J Radiol* 1999;*172*:1541–1546.

Lemmer ER, Spearman CWN, Krige JEJ, Millar AJW, Bornman PC, Terblanche J, Kahn D. The management of biliary complications following orthotopic liver transplantation. *S Afr J Surg* 1997;*35*:77–81.

Macedo G, Maia JC, Gomes A, Teixeira A, Ribeiro T. The role of transjugular liver biopsy in a liver transplant center. *J Clin Gastroenterol* 1999;*29*:155–157.

Montalvo BM, Yrizarry JM, Casillas VJ, et al. Percutaneous sclerotherapy of lymphoceles related to renal transplantation. *J Vasc Int Radiol* 1996;*7*:117–123.

Neimatallah MA, Dong Q, Schoenberg SO, Cho KJ, Prince MR. Magnetic resonance imaging in renal transplantation. *J Mag Res Im* 1999;*10*:357–368.

Nelson HA, Gilfeather M, Holman JM, Nelson EW, Yoon HC. Gadolinium-enhanced breathhold three-dimensional time-of-flight renal MR angiography in the evaluation of potential renal donors. *J Vasc Interven Radiol* 199;*10*:175–181.

Nelson NL, Largen PS, Stratta RJ, et al. Pancreas allograft rejection: Correlation of transduodenal core biopsy with Doppler resistive index. *Radiology* 1996;*200*:91–94.

Newman-Sanders AP, Gedroyc WG, Al-Kutoubi MA, Koo C, Taube D. The use of expandable metal stents in transplant renal artery stenosis. *Clin Radiol* 1995;*50*:245–250.

Nghiem HV. Imaging of hepatic transplantation. *Radiol Clin North Am* 1998;*36*:429–443.

Oremonde DG, de Boer WB, Kierath A, Bell R, Shilkin KB, House AK, Jeffrey GP, Reed WD. Banff schema for grading liver allograft rejection: Utility in clinical practice. *Liver Transpl Surg* 1999;*5*:261–268.

Patel BK, Garvin PJ, Aridge DL, Chenoweth JL, Markivee CR. Fluid collections developing after pancreatic transplantation: Radiologic evaluation and intervention. *Radiology* 1991;*181*:215–220.

Patenaude YG, DuBois J, Sinsky AB, et al. Liver transplantation: Review of the literature: Part 2: Vascular and biliary complications. *Can Assoc Radiol* 1997;*48*:231–242.

Poles MA, Martin P. Routine endoscopy in liver transplant candidates: Is it indicated? *Am J Gastroenterol* 1999;*94*:871–872.

Porayko MK, Knodo M, Steers JL. Liver transplantation: Late complications of the biliary tract and their management. *Semin Liver Dis* 1995;*15*:139–155.

Pozniak MA, Balison DJ, Lee FT, Tambeaux RH, Uehling DT, Moon TD. CT angiography of potential renal transplant donors. *RadioGraphics* 1998;*18*:565–587.

Rubin R, Munoz SJ. Clinicopathologic features of late hepatic dysfunction in orthotopic liver transplants. *Hum Pathol* 1993;*24*:643–651.

Siegelman ES, Outwater EK. MR imaging techniques of the liver. *Radiol Clin North Am* 1998;*36*: 263–284.

Taylor HM, Ros PR. Hepatic imaging: An overview. *Radiol Clin North Am* 1998;*36*:237–245.

Todo S, Demetris AJ, Van Thiel D, et al. Primary non-function of hepatic allografts with preexisting fatty infiltration. *Transplantation* 1989;*47*:903–905.

Yang MD, Wu CC, Chen HC, Liu TJ, Chi CS, Ho YJ, P'Eng FK. Biliary complications in long-term recipients of reduced size liver transplants. *Transpl Proc* 1996;*28*:1680–1681.

Zajko AB, Sheng R, Bron K, Reyes J, Nour B, Tzakis A. Percutaneous transluminal angioplasty of venous anastomotic stenoses complicating liver transplantation: Intermediate-term results. *J Vasc Int Radiol* 1994;*5*:121–126.

Zaman A, Hapke R, Flora K, Rosen H, Benner K. Prevalence of upper and lower gastrointestinal tract findings in liver transplant candidates undergoing screening endoscopic evaluation. *Am J Gastroenterol* 1999;*94*:895–899.

RECOMMENDED WEBSITES

Centers for Disease Control and Prevention: *www.cdc.gov*

DOT (Division of Transplantation, USA): *http.//www.hrsa.dhhs.gov/osp/dot/*

FDA Center for Biologics Evaluation and Research: *http://www.fda.gov/cber/publications.htm*

Immune Tolerance Network: *http://www.immunetolerance.org*

International Pancreas Transplant Registry: *http://www.umn.edu.itpr*

National Institute of Diabetes and Digestive and Kidney Disease: *http://www.niddk.nih.gov/*

National Institute of Diabetes and Digestive and Kidney Disease Liver Transplantation Database: *http://www.niddk.nih.gov/*

United Network for Organ Sharing: *http://www.unos.org*

United States Department of Health and Human Services—National Organ and Tissue Donation Initiative: *http://www.organdonor.gov*

United States Renal Data System: *http://www.med.umich.edu/usrds/*

Index